Guide to Assessment Scales in Schizophrenia

3rd edition

Editor
Richard Keefe

Contributors

Jean Addington, George Awad, Anthony S David, Donald Goff, Philip D Harvey, Michael Kraus, Julie Kreyenbuhl, Jonathan C Lee, Stephen Marder, Joseph P McEvoy, Ashwin A Patkar, Mark Taylor, Joseph Ventura

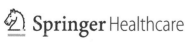 **Springer** Healthcare

Published by Springer Healthcare Ltd, 236 Gray's Inn Road, London, WC1X 8HB, UK.

www.springerhealthcare.com

ISBN 978-1-908517-52-4

British Library Cataloguing-in-Publication Data.

A catalogue record for this book is available from the British Library.

Although every effort has been made to ensure that drug doses and other information are presented accurately in this publication, the ultimate responsibility rests with the prescribing physician. Neither the publisher nor the authors can be held responsible for errors or for any consequences arising from the use of the information contained herein. Any product mentioned in this publication should be used in accordance with the prescribing information prepared by the manufacturers. No claims or endorsements are made for any drug or compound at present under clinical investigation.

Project editor: Tamsin Curtis
Designer: Joe Harvey
Artworker: Sissan Mollerfors
Production: Marina Maher
Printed in Great Britain by Latimer Trend & Company Ltd.

Contents

Author biographies

Editor

Richard Keefe, PhD, is Professor of Psychiatry and Behavioral Sciences at Duke University Medical Center in Durham, North Carolina. He received his BA from Princeton University and his PhD in clinical psychology from New York University. His research is primarily devoted to understanding cognitive dysfunction and its treatment in patients with schizophrenia and related disorders, including those at high risk for schizophrenia. Dr Keefe has had a leadership role in several large National Institute of Mental Health studies including the CATIE, MATRICS, TURNS, and TENETS projects. He has authored more than 160 peer-reviewed scientific papers and two books. He serves on the editorial boards of several journals, including *Schizophrenia Research, Schizophrenia Bulletin,* and *Innovations in Clinical Neuroscience,* and is Associate Editor of *Psychological Medicine.* He is President of the International Society for CNS Clinical Trials and Methodology for 2012–2014. He is the Founder and CEO of NeuroCog Trials, Inc. He is a Co-Principal Investigator and Director of the Neurocognitive Core for the Translational and Clinical Research Neuroscience project at the Institute of Mental Health in Singapore.

Contributors

Jean Addington, PhD, is Professor of Psychiatry at the University of Calgary and holds the Alberta Centennial Mental Health Research Chair and the Novartis Chair for Schizophrenia Research. Professor Addington graduated from The University of Calgary, Alberta, Canada. She has authored and contributed to a broad range of international publications and books on schizophrenia and other psychotic disorders and was one of the developers of the Calgary Depression Scale for Schizophrenia. Professor Addington's research interests are in early detection and intervention in psychosis, specifically the examination of predictors of conversion to psychosis and the development of psychosocial interventions for those at clinical high risk of psychosis.

George Awad, MBBCh, PhD, FRCP(C), is currently Professor Emeritus of Psychiatry at the University of Toronto and is on the faculty of the Institute of Medical Science in the School of Graduate Studies. He is also the Chief of the Department of Psychiatry at Humber River Regional Hospital, Toronto, Ontario. Dr Awad is the recipient of the Tanenbaum Distinguished Scientist Award in Schizophrenia Research. He is a past President of the Canadian College of Neuropsychopharmacology. Recently, he was awarded the College Medal for meritorious contributions in psychopharmacology research, teaching and services. Dr Awad was the Founding President of the International Society for CNS Clinical Trials and Methodology for three years. Dr Awad continues to be extensively involved in training, research, and lecturing nationally and internationally. Dr Awad has published extensively including a number of books, the most recent of which is *Quality of Life Impairment in Schizophrenia, Mood and Anxiety Disorders.*

Anthony S David, MD, MSc, FRCP, FRCPsych, is a clinical psychiatrist and academic currently working at the Maudsley Hospital, and Institute of Psychiatry, King's College London. He graduated in medicine from Glasgow University and trained in neurology before entering psychiatry. He has been Professor of Cognitive Neuropsychiatry since 1996 and is editor of the *Journal of Cognitive Neuropsychiatry* and has authored and contributed to over 400 peer-reviewed scientific articles in the field of schizophrenia, neuropsychiatry, neuropsychology and brain imaging, and has published several books, including *Insight and Psychosis: Awareness of Illness in Schizophrenia and Related Disorders.* He has a long-standing interest in schizophrenia as well as neuropsychology and brain imaging.

Donald Goff, MD, is Director of the Schizophrenia Program at Massachusetts General Hospital and Professor of Psychiatry at Harvard Medical School in Boston. Dr Goff earned his medical degree at the UCLA School of Medicine, Los Angeles, California, and completed his internship in Internal Medicine at Cedars-Sinai Medical Center in Los Angeles and his residency in Psychiatry at Massachusetts General Hospital in Boston, Massachusetts. His research fellowship in psychopharmacology was completed at Tufts-New England Medical Center in Boston. Dr Goff has published over 200 articles concerning schizophrenia and related topics. He is director of a clinical research program of 12 investigators integrating pharmacology, cognitive behavioral therapy, neuroimaging, and genetics to enhance understanding of the pathophysiology of schizophrenia and to develop new treatments. Dr Goff is the recipient of the Kempf Award for Mentorship in Biological Psychiatry from the American Psychiatric Association, the Wayne Fenton, MD, Award for Exceptional Clinical Care, and the Stanley Dean Award for Research in Schizophrenia from the American College of Psychiatrists.

Philip D Harvey, PhD, is Professor of Psychiatry at the University of Miami Miller School of Medicine. He is the author of over 800 scientific papers and abstracts and he has written over 50 book chapters. His work has been cited more than 500 times per year for the past decade, with over 1500 citations of his work in 2010. He has given more than 1800 presentations at scientific conferences and medical education events. He has edited five and written four books on topics of psychological assessment, schizophrenia, and aging. He has received a number of awards and is a member of the American Psychological Association, the American College of Neuropsychopharmacology (Fellow), the International College of Neuropsychopharmacology (Fellow), the Society for Research in Psychopathology (Founding Member), the Society for Biological Psychiatry, International Neuropsychological Society, the Schizophrenia International Research Society (Founding Director), and the International Society for Clinical Trials and Methodology (Founding Member). His research has focused on cognition and functioning and he has written extensively on aging in schizophrenia, functional impairments in severe mental illness, the cognitive effects of typical and atypical antipsychotics, as well as studying the effects of cognitive enhancing agents in various conditions, including schizophrenia, dementia, affective disorders, and traumatic brain injury.

Michael S Kraus, MA, is an Associate in Research in the Department of Psychiatry and Behavioral Science, Duke University Medical Center, Durham, North Carolina. He graduated from Grinnell

College, Iowa, before attending the Yale Neurobiology graduate program at Yale University, New Haven, Connecticut. Michael Kraus has authored and contributed to several international publications. His principal research interests include cognitive deficits in schizophrenia and auditory and emotional processing deficits in schizophrenia.

Julie Kreyenbuhl, PharmD, PhD, is a research investigator with the US Department of Veterans Affairs Capitol Healthcare Network Mental Illness Research, Education, and Clinical Center and a member of the faculty at the University of Maryland School of Medicine, Department of Psychiatry, Division of Services Research. She completed her clinical pharmacy training at Mercer University College of Pharmacy and Health Sciences in Atlanta, Georgia, in 1993 and received a PhD in Pharmaceutical Health Services Research from the University of Maryland School of Pharmacy in Baltimore, Maryland, in 1999. She completed a post-doctoral fellowship at the Maryland Psychiatric Research Center in Baltimore, Maryland, in 2000. Dr Kreyenbuhl has authored or co-authored over 50 publications in peer-reviewed journals and has contributed extensively to the development of evidence-based treatment guidelines for schizophrenia. Her current research focuses on testing the effectiveness of computer technology-based interventions for individuals with serious mental illnesses in the areas of enhancing adherence to and providing education about the medication side effects of antipsychotic medications.

Jonathan C Lee, MD, is the Associate Medical Director of the Farley Center at Williamsburg Place in Virginia. He is a graduate of the Massachusetts Institute of Technology, and the University of Virginia School of Medicine. In 2010 he completed a combined residency in internal medicine and psychiatry at Duke University Medical Center in Durham, North Carolina, serving as Chief Resident of Medicine and Psychiatry from 2009 to 2010. He is Board Certified with the American Board of Internal Medicine and is Board Eligible with the American Board of Psychiatry and Neurology as well as the American Board of Addiction Medicine. Dr Lee is a member of the Association of Medicine and Psychiatry, American College of Physicians, American Psychiatric Association, American Academy of Addiction Psychiatry, and American Society of Addiction Medicine. He has authored and contributed to literature in psychosomatic medicine and addiction medicine. He has conducted clinical research in collaboration with the Duke Addictions Program in Durham, North Carolina.

Stephen R Marder, MD, is Professor and Director of the Section on Psychosis at the UCLA Semel Institute for Neuroscience and Director of the VISN 22 Mental Illness Research, Education Clinical Center (MIRECC) for the Department of Veterans Affairs. He graduated from the University of Pennsylvania and received his medical degree from the State University of New York, Buffalo. After an internship at Denver General Hospital he completed a residency at the University of Southern California. He was a Clinical Associate in the Biological Psychiatry Branch at the National Institute of Mental Health from 1975–1977, then in 1977 he joined the staff at the Brentwood VA Medical Center and the faculty at UCLA. Dr Marder's research has focused on the drug treatment of schizophrenia and the pharmacology of antipsychotic drugs. He has authored or co-authored more than 200 journal articles and chapters based on research. Dr Marder has received the Exemplary Psychiatrist Award from the National Alliance for the Mentally Ill, the Stanley Dean Research Award of the American College of Psychiatry, the Alexander Gralnick Award from the American Psychiatric Association, the Outstanding Achievement Award of the Southern California Psychiatric Society, and the Kempf Award from the American Psychiatric Association. He is listed in *The Best Doctors in America* and *America's Top Doctors*.

Joseph P McEvoy, MD, is currently Professor of Psychiatry and Behavioral Sciences at Duke University, Durham, North Carolina. He graduated from Vanderbilt Medical School in 1973 and took two years of residency in Internal Medicine at the University of Utah Hospitals, and then returned to Vanderbilt to complete a psychiatry residency. He has served on the faculties of Vanderbilt University and the University of Pittsburgh and as Co-Principal Investigator and Project Medical Officer for the CATIE Schizophrenia trials and the Schizophrenia Trials Network, and he chaired the Metabolic Working Group for these trials. He has authored more than 150 refereed publications, two books, and numerous book chapters. He is a Distinguished Fellow of the American Psychiatric Association.

Ashwin A Patkar, MD, MRCPsych, completed his medical school education at G S Medical College in Mumbai, India, his MRCPsych from the Royal College of Psychiatrists, England, and a Neuropharmacology degree from University of Nottingham, England. He completed his psychiatry residency at Thomas Jefferson University Philadelphia (1995–1997) and was the Director of Biological Psychiatry and Clinical Trials at Thomas Jefferson University. Since 2004, Dr Patkar has been an Associate Professor of Psychiatry and Medical Director of Duke Addictions Programs at Duke University Medical Center, Durham, North Carolina. He is Board Certified in Psychiatry with additional Certification in Addiction Psychiatry, Addiction Medicine, and Pain Medicine. Dr Patkar has authored/co-authored over 175 peer-reviewed publications and has given over 200 presentations and invited lectures at national and international meetings. He is a member of two peer-reviewed journal editorial boards and is an active member of several national and international medical societies. His principal area of interest is addiction.

Mark Taylor, BSc (Hons), MBBS, FRCPsych, FRANZCP, is a full-time clinician and consultant adult psychiatrist and was appointed in 2008 to set up an intensive home treatment service for the city of Edinburgh, which won the Royal College of Psychiatrists' Team of the Year award in 2010. In 2011, his team also won the Scottish Health Awards in the 'Care at Home' category; and were shortlisted finalists in the *Health Service Journal* Innovation in Mental Healthcare awards. Dr Taylor obtained his medical degree from University College London and then gained experience in neurology and general medicine at Guys Hospital, London, before training in psychiatry at the Maudsley Hospital and Institute of Psychiatry, London and the University of Edinburgh. He has previously worked as a consultant psychiatrist in both Glasgow, Scotland, and Melbourne, Australia. Dr Taylor is an Honorary Clinical Senior Lecturer at the University of Edinburgh and University of Glasgow and teaches under- and postgraduate medics. Dr Taylor publishes peer-reviewed academic papers, and he won the Scottish Mental Health Research Network prize in 2010. He delivers invited national and international lectures regularly.

Joseph Ventura is a member of the UCLA Department of Psychiatry Faculty, the Director of the Functional Outcome and Symptom Assessment Core of the UCLA Center for Cognition and Emotion in Schizophrenia, and the Director of the Cognitive Remediation program at the UCLA Aftercare Research Program. Dr Ventura has been successful in obtaining independent research funding from the National Institute of Mental Health, the National Alliance for Research on Schizophrenia, and the pharmaceutical industry. Dr Ventura has published over 100 peer-reviewed journal articles, book chapters, and scientific abstracts. His research has concentrated on predictors of course and functional outcome in the early phase of schizophrenia including stressful life events, positive and negative symptoms, disorganization, insight, neurocognition, and social cognition. Areas of recent interest include factors that are associated with recovery from schizophrenia and the development of interview-based assessments of cognitive functioning. Dr Ventura played a major role in the development and publication of methods for standardized diagnostic and psychiatric symptom assessment training and quality assurance. He has set standards for achieving and maintaining high levels of inter-rater reliability aimed at preventing 'rater drift.' Dr Ventura has conducted numerous workshops and lectured nationally and internationally on topics such as neurocognition, social cognition, diagnosis, symptoms, structured assessment, and functional outcome.

Preface

The aim of this guide is to provide clinicians with a single volume to aid in the comprehensive assessment of patients with schizophrenia. It is meant for early phase clinicians as a means to learn the best scales to use in the assessment of various aspects of the illness and for established clinicians as an organizing resource that will enable them to have direct access to many assessment instruments housed in one book.

In the past, rating scales for patients with schizophrenia had been viewed as the domain of researchers or clinical trialists willing to sacrifice patient interaction for standardization of data collection. However, the assessment instruments in this book are being used with increased frequency due to a variety of changes in the administration of care in clinical psychiatry. The use of integrated care pathways, the burgeoning emphasis on payment by results, and the pursuit of evidence-based practice principles encourage the use of standardized instruments in mental health care. Many clinicians find that a structured approach to the assessment of their patients not only helps to organize their patient evaluations, but also helps them keep track of changes across time especially with regard to treatment response. Further, an understanding of how a patient fits within the spectrum of similarly diagnosed patients can have important treatment implications. Finally, rating scales can help a clinician consider broad aspects of a patient's illness that are not usually fully evaluated, especially in areas where his or her training may be limited, such as cognition.

We have included scales measuring all of the crucial aspects of schizophrenia: symptoms, including positive and negative symptoms; depression and suicidality; cognition, including interview-based rating scales and performance-based assessments; functional outcomes such as work function, social function, and independent living; quality of life; side effects of antipsychotic treatment; insight; treatment adherence; substance abuse; and medical comorbidities.

The authors of the chapters were selected on the basis of the international renown of the high quality of their research and clinical work in the specific areas they cover. We are delighted that due to the importance of this work and the necessity of this resource, many of the true leaders of research and clinical work in schizophrenia agreed to participate.

In many cases, the specific rating scale is included in the guide. Due to copyright restrictions of some of the instruments, this was not permitted for all of the rating scales. However, in these cases we have included the source where the specific scale can be obtained.

We hope that this guide is beneficial to those clinicians who utilize it and to the patients who are assessed with the instruments herein.

Richard Keefe, PhD
Durham, North Carolina, USA

1. Symptom rating scales in schizophrenia

Joseph Ventura and Stephen Marder

Standardized psychiatric symptom rating scales were originally developed for research purposes such as in pharmacological clinical trials; however, they can be used by clinicians to reliably document symptoms. Rating scales can be useful tools for establishing the initial levels of symptoms and assessing the response to an intervention. The most useful symptom rating scales provide clinical interview questions with follow-up probes to be used during a 20- to 30-minute semi-structured interview to assess psychopathology. The clinician should draw on all sources of information including direct observation of patient behavior, reports from the patient, observations from nurses, and reports from the patient's family. Psychiatric symptom rating scales differ in the breadth of type of symptoms that can be assessed, but generally use the same format. Each scale has an instructional manual with symptom definitions, a rating scale with anchor point definitions, and a set of standardized interview questions with suggested follow-up probes. The anchor points of a rating scale describe the severity of a particular symptom; for example, on a scale of 1–7, 1 being 'not present,' which represents the absence of psychopathology, ratings of 2 or 3 are considered mild, clinically sub-threshold, or generally within normal limits, while ratings of 4 or 5 are considered at a moderate level and therefore clinically significant. Ratings of 6 or 7 are considered a severe level of psychopathology.

The proper reference group for conducting symptom rating assessments is a group of individuals who are not psychiatric patients, who are living and working in the community, who are not receiving psychiatric medication and, who are relatively free of psychiatric symptoms. As the clinician evaluates patients, he or she should have in mind a group of individuals who are able to function either at work or school, socially or as a homemaker, and at levels appropriate to the person's age and socioeconomic status. Clinicians assessing symptoms should not use other psychiatric patients previously interviewed, especially those with severe symptoms, as the reference standard because this approach will systematically bias ratings toward lower scores. If symptom ratings are to be used for monitoring symptoms over time then selecting an appropriate period or interval for rating symptoms is important; for example, just prior to hospitalization versus following a reasonable course of treatment.

Good interviewing skills, interpersonal rapport, sensitivity to the patient's mental state, and empathy are of paramount importance in obtaining valid ratings of symptoms. The use of empathy

R. Keefe (ed.), *Guide to Assessment Scales in Schizophrenia*,
DOI: 10.1007/978-1-908517-71-5_1,
© Springer Healthcare, a part of Springer Science+Business Media 2012

is critical in helping a patient express difficult and possibly embarrassing experiences. An all too common phenomenon in clinical assessment is the denial or minimization of psychiatric symptoms. For example, patients may deny hearing voices yet can be observed to be whispering under their breath as if in response to a voice. Patients deny their symptoms for a variety of reasons, including fear of being committed, restricted to staying in a hospital, or having their medication increased. Simply recording a patient's negative response to symptom scale items, if denial or distortion is present, will result in invalid and unreliable data. Occasionally, at the time of the interview, the interviewer will have information about the symptoms that the patient is denying. The use of a mild confrontation technique is permissible in an attempt to encourage a patient to disclose accurate symptom information. When an interviewer suspects that a patient may be denying symptoms, soliciting and utilizing information from other sources is absolutely essential in rating symptom psychopathology.

Positive symptom scales

Positive symptoms in schizophrenia include:
- hallucinations (perceptual abnormalities) in one of five senses (auditory, visual, tactile, olfactory, or gustatory);
- delusions (false beliefs), most commonly persecutory, referential, grandiose, or somatic; and
- disorders of thought (speech abnormalities), indicated by speech that is tangential, circumstantial, shows derailment, or is incoherent.

These symptoms are primarily found in the Positive and Negative Syndrome Scale (PANSS) [1], the Brief Psychiatric Rating Scale (BPRS) [2], and the Scale for the Assessment of Positive Symptoms (SAPS) [3], but these instruments also contain negative symptom items particularly the PANSS, which was developed with the goal of giving similar weight to both positive and negative symptoms. If a clinician is interested in comprehensive treatment of a psychotic disorder, then specialized scales for the assessment of negative symptoms should be used adjunctively.

Positive and Negative Syndrome Scale

The PANSS [1] contains 30 items of which seven were chosen to constitute a Positive Symptom Scale, seven items in a Negative Symptom Scale, and the remaining sixteen in a General Psychopathology Scale. The PANSS rates psychopathology on a scale from 1 to 7, 1 being 'absent' and 7 being 'extreme,' through evaluation and observation of:
- behavior (eg, tension, mannerisms and posturing, excitement, and blunting of affect);
- interpersonal behavior during the interview (eg, poor rapport, uncooperativeness, hostility, and impaired attention);
- cognitive–verbal processes (eg, conceptual disorganization, stereotyped thinking, and lack of spontaneity and flow of conversation);
- expressed thought content (eg, grandiosity, somatic concern, guilt feelings, and delusions); and

- response to structured interviewing (eg, disorientation, anxiety, depression, and difficulty in abstract thinking).

A unique feature of the PANSS is the comprehensive evaluation of abstract reasoning. The PANSS contains questions on concept formulation (eg, "How are a train and bus alike?") and proverb interpretation, which are varied in content when using the PANSS for repeated assessment.

For further discussion on the PANSS see Chapter 7.

Brief Psychiatric Rating Scale – 24-item version

The 24-item version of the BPRS [2] contains symptom items that yield a comprehensive rating of major psychiatric symptoms such as anxiety, depression, suicidality, hostility, delusions, hallucinations, disorganized speech, mania, disorientation, and bizarre behavior. One unique feature of the BPRS is the inclusion of an item for assessment of suicidality. Each BPRS item is rated on increasing levels of psychopathology ranging from 1 to 7, with 1 being 'absent' to 7 being 'extremely severe.' The 24-item version of the BPRS contains interview questions, symptom definitions, specific anchor points for rating symptoms, and a detailed 'how to' section for dilemmas that arise in rating psychopathology. The easily understood definitions and anchor point definitions assist the clinician in sensitively eliciting and rating the severity of psychiatric symptoms. The BPRS enables the clinician to conduct a high-quality interview for eliciting and rating the severity of mood and psychotic symptoms in individuals who are often inarticulate or who deny their illness. Four sample BPRS items were selected to provide the clinician with an opportunity to determine the potential usefulness of the full 24-item BPRS for evaluation of psychiatric symptoms. Three of the selected BPRS items are positive symptoms, unusual thought content, hallucinations, and conceptual disorganization, which are most likely to be exhibited in psychiatric patients who are acutely psychotic. The suicidality item from the BPRS is provided because of the clinical relevance for evaluating this potentially lethal behavior in psychiatric patients who are presenting with acute symptoms or during routine evaluation (Figure 1.1) [2].

Scale for the Assessment of Positive Symptoms

The SAPS [3] is a 35-item instrument designed to assess all of the key positive symptoms of psychosis that principally occur in schizophrenia. The SAPS is intended to serve as a complementary instrument to the Scale for the Assessment of Negative Symptoms (SANS). Positive symptoms assessed by the SAPS include hallucinations, delusions, bizarre behavior (including inappropriate affect), and formal thought disorder (disorganization of speech). The SAPS is the most comprehensive scale for the assessment of positive formal thought disorder so the clinician should begin this assessment interview by talking with the patient on a relatively neutral topic for 5–10 minutes in order to observe the patient's manner of speaking and responding. The last symptom item in each major domain of positive symptoms is an overall global rating. This should be a true global rating based on taking into account both the content and the severity of the various types of symptoms observed. Each SAPS item is accompanied by a complete definition as well as detailed anchoring criteria for all six rating points ranging from 0 ('absent') to 5 ('severe').

Figure 1.1 Brief Psychiatric Rating Scale – 24-item version

Conceptual disorganization

Degree to which speech is confused, disconnected, vague or disorganized. Rate tangentiality, circumstantiality, sudden topic shifts, incoherence, derailment, blocking, neologisms, and other speech disorders. Do not rate content of speech.

1 = Not present

2 = Very mild
Peculiar use of words or rambling but speech is comprehensible.

3 = Mild
Speech a bit hard to understand or make sense of due to tangentiality, circumstantiality, or sudden topic shifts.

4 = Moderate
Speech difficult to understand due to tangentiality, circumstantiality, idiosyncratic speech, or topic shifts on many occasions **or** 1 or 2 instances of incoherent phrases.

5 = Moderately severe
Speech difficult to understand due to circumstantiality, tangentiality, neologisms, blocking, or topic shifts most of the time **or** 3–5 instances of incoherent phrases.

6 = Severe
Speech is incomprehensible due to severe impairments most of the time. Many items in this scale cannot be rated by self report alone.

7 = Extremely severe
Speech is incomprehensible throughout interview.

Suicidality

Expressed desire, intent or actions to harm or kill self.

Questions to ask patient:
- Have you felt that life wasn't worth living?
- Have you thought about harming or killing yourself?
- Have you felt tired of living or as though you would be better off dead?
- Have you ever felt like ending it all?

If patient reports suicidal ideation, ask the following:
- How often have you thought about [use patient's description]?
- Did/Do you have a specific plan?

1 = Not present

2 = Very mild
Occasional feelings of being tired of living. No overt suicidal thoughts.

3 = Mild
Occasional suicidal thoughts without intent or specific plan **or** they feel they would be better off dead.

4 = Moderate
Suicidal thoughts frequent without intent or plan.

5 = Moderately severe
Many fantasies of suicide by various methods. May seriously consider making an attempt with specific time and plan **or** impulsive suicide attempt using nonlethal method or in full view of potential saviors.

6 = Severe
Clearly wants to kill self. Searches for appropriate means and time, **or** potentially serious suicide attempt with patient knowledge of possible rescue.

7 = Extremely severe
Specific suicidal plan and intent (eg, "As soon as this happens I will do it by doing X"), **or** suicide attempt characterized by plan patient thought was lethal or attempt in secluded environment.

(continues opposite).

Figure 1.1 Brief Psychiatric Rating Scale – 24-item version (continued)

Unusual thought content

Unusual, odd, strange or bizarre thought content. Rate the degree of unusualness, not the degree of disorganization of speech. Delusions are patently absurd, clearly false or bizarre ideas that are expressed with full conviction. Consider the patient to have full conviction if they have acted as though the delusional belief were true. Ideas of reference/persecution can be differentiated from delusions in that ideas are expressed with much doubt and contain more elements of reality. Include thought insertion, withdrawal, and broadcast. Include grandiose, somatic and persecutory delusions even if rated elsewhere. Note: if somatic concern, guilt, suspiciousness, or grandiosity are rated 6 or 7 due to delusions, then unusual thought content must be rated 4 or above.

Questions to ask patient:
- Have you been receiving any special messages from people or from the way things are arranged around you?
- Have you seen any references to yourself on TV or in the newspapers?
- Can anyone read your mind?
- Do you have a special relationship with God?
- Is anything like electricity, X-rays, or radio waves affecting you?
- Are thoughts put into your head that are not your own?
- Have you felt that you were under the control of another person or force?

If patient reports any odd ideas/delusions, ask the following:
- How often do you think about [use patient's description]?
- Have you told anyone about these experiences?
- How do you explain the things that have been happening [specify with examples from patient]?

1 = Not present

2 = Very mild
Ideas of reference (people may stare or may laugh at them), ideas of persecution (people may mistreat them). Unusual beliefs in psychic powers, spirits, UFOs, or unrealistic beliefs in one's own abilities. Not strongly held. Some doubt.

3 = Mild
Same as 2, but degree of reality distortion is more severe as indicated by highly unusual ideas or greater conviction. Content may be typical of delusions (even bizarre), but without full conviction. The delusion does not seem to have fully formed, but is considered as one possible explanation for an unusual experience.

4 = Moderate
Delusion present but no preoccupation or functional impairment. May be an encapsulated delusion or a firmly endorsed absurd belief about past delusional circumstances.

5 = Moderately severe
Full delusion(s) present with some preoccupation **or** some areas of functioning disrupted by delusional thinking.

6 = Severe
Full delusion(s) present with much preoccupation **or** many areas of functioning are disrupted by delusional thinking.

7 = Extremely severe
Full delusion(s) present with almost total preoccupation **or** most areas of functioning are disrupted by delusional thinking.

(continues overleaf).

Figure 1.1 Brief Psychiatric Rating Scale – 24-item version (continued)

Hallucinations

Reports of perceptual experiences in the absence of relevant external stimuli. When rating degree to which functioning is disrupted by hallucinations, include preoccupation with the content and experience of the hallucinations, as well as functioning disrupted by acting out on the hallucinatory content (eg, engaging in deviant behavior due to command hallucinations). Include thoughts aloud ('gedankenlautwerden') or pseudohallucinations (eg, hears a voice inside head) if a voice quality is present.

Questions to ask patient:
- Do you ever seem to hear your name being called?
- Have you heard any sounds or people talking to you or about you when there has been nobody around?

If the patient hears voices, ask the following:
- What does the voice/voices say?
- Did it have a voice quality?
- Do you ever have visions or see things that others do not see?
- What about smell odors that others do not smell?

If the patient reports hallucinations, ask the following:
- Have these experiences interfered with your ability to perform your usual activities/work?
- How do you explain them?
- How often do they occur?

1 = Not present

2 = Very mild
While resting or going to sleep, sees visions, smells odors, or hears voices, sounds, or whispers in the absence of external stimulation, but no impairment in functioning.

3 = Mild
While in a clear state of consciousness, hears a voice calling the subjects name, experiences nonverbal auditory hallucinations (eg, sounds or whispers), formless visual hallucinations, or has sensory experiences in the presence of a modality relevant stimulus (eg, visual illusions) infrequently (eg, 1–2 times per week) and with no functional impairment.

4 = Moderate
Occasional verbal, visual, gustatory, olfactory, or tactile hallucinations with no functional impairment **or** non verbal auditory hallucinations/visual illusions more than infrequently or with impairment.

5 = Moderately severe
Experiences daily hallucinations **or** some areas of functioning are disrupted by hallucinations.

6 = Severe
Experiences verbal or visual hallucinations several times a day **or** many areas of functioning are disrupted by these hallucinations.

7 = Extremely severe
Persistent verbal or visual hallucinations throughout the day **or** most areas of functioning are disrupted by these hallucinations.

(continued). Data from Ventura et al [2]. © 1993, reproduced with permission from John Wiley and Sons.

Figure 1.2 4-Item Negative Symptom Assessment

Restricted speech quantity	1. Normal speech quantity. 2. Minimal reduction in quantity; may be extreme side of normal. 3. Speech quantity is reduced, but more obtained with minimal prodding. 4. Flow of speech is maintained only by regularly prodding. 5. Responses usually limited to a few words, and/or detail is only obtained by prodding or bribing. 6. Responses usually nonverbal or limited to 1 or 2 words despite efforts to elicit more. 7. Not ratable.
Emotion: reduced range (specify time frame for this assessment)	1. Normal range of emotion. 2. Minimal reduction in range; may be extreme side of normal. 3. Range seems restricted relative to a normal person, but during the specified time period subject convincingly reports at least four emotions. 4. Subject convincingly identifies two or three emotional experiences. 5. Subject can convincingly identify only one emotional experience. 6. Subject reports little or no emotional range. 7. Not ratable.
Reduced social drive	1. Normal social drive. 2. Minimal reduction in social drive; may be extreme side of normal. 3. Desire for social interactions seems somewhat reduced. 4. Obvious reduction in desire to initiate social contacts, but a number of social contacts are initiated each week. 5. Marked reduction in desire to initiate social contacts, but a few contacts are maintained at subject's initiation (as with family). 6. No desire to initiate any social interactions. 7. Not ratable.
Reduced interests	1. Normal interests. 2. Minimal reduction in interests; may be extreme side of normal. 3. Range of interests and/or commitment to them seems diminished. 4. Range of interests is clearly diminished and subject is not particularly committed to interests held. 5. Only one or two interests reported, and these pursued superficially. 6. Little or nothing stimulates interest. 7. Not ratable.

Data from Alphs et al [7]. Reproduced with permission from Matrix Medical Communications.

Negative symptom scales

Negative symptoms in schizophrenia include blunted or restricted affect, alogia, asociality, anhedonia, and avolition [4]. Some of these items are included in instruments that measure positive symptoms, particularly the PANSS, which was developed with the goal of giving similar weight to both positive and negative symptoms. However, if a clinician is focused on treating negative symptoms, primarily positive symptom scales may not provide all of the coverage that will permit an adequate evaluation. For this reason, specialized scales for negative symptoms may be the best choice.

Scale for the Assessment of Negative Symptoms

The SANS [5] is a 25-item instrument that is widely used to measure five negative symptoms domains including:

- affective flattening (blunted affect);
- alogia;
- avolition and apathy;
- asociality; and
- attention.

Each SANS item is accompanied by a complete definition as well as detailed anchoring criteria for all six rating points ranging from 0 ('absent') to 5 ('severe'). The SANS is the most comprehensive standardized scale for the assessment of negative symptoms. Recent versions have eliminated items that were included in the original instrument, such as inappropriate affect (from affective flattening), poverty of content of speech (from alogia), the patient's subjective impression of his or her negative symptoms, and attentional impairment. These items are currently considered to be associated with positive symptoms in schizophrenia or in the case of the patient's subjective impression, prove difficult to rate reliably.

Negative Symptom Assessment Scale

The Negative Symptom Assessment Scale (NSA) [6] is a 23-item instrument and includes a global rating that assesses the five primary domains of negative symptoms. A revised 16-item version, the NSA-16, is considered easier to use and is most commonly used in clinical trials. An important advantage of the NSA-16 is that the asociality–avolition component more sensitively differentiates between actual negative symptoms and the patient's intentional behavior. For example, the NSA-16 measures a reduced sense of purpose and reduced social drive as negative symptom assessment items. A recently proposed four-item version of the NSA-16 may be particularly useful for clinical settings (Figure 1.2) [7].

Rating scales for depressive symptoms and suicidality are discussed in detail in Chapter 2.

References

1   Kay SR, Fiszbein A, Opler LA. The Positive and Negative Syndrome Scale (PANSS) for schizophrenia. *Schizophrenia Bull*. 1987;13:261-276.
2   Ventura J, Lukoff D, Nuechterlein KH, Liberman RP, Green MF, Shaner A. Brief Psychiatric Rating Scale (BPRS) expanded version (4.0): scales, anchor points, and administration manual. *Int J Methods Psych Res*. 1993;3:227-243.
3   Andreasen NC. *The Scale for the Assessment of Positive Symptoms (SAPS)*. Iowa City, IA: The University of Iowa; 1984.
4   Kirkpatrick B, Fenton WS, Carpenter WT, Jr, Marder SR. The NIMH-MATRICS consensus statement on negative symptoms. *Schizophr Bull*. 2006;32:214-219.
5   Andreasen NC. Scale for the Assessment of Negative Symptoms (SANS). *Br J Psychiatry*. 1983;154:672-676.
6   Axelrod BN, Goldman RS, Woodard JL, Alphs LD. Factor structure of the negative symptom assessment. *Psychiatry Res*. 1994;52:173-179.
7   Alphs L, Morlock R, Coon C, van Willigenburg A, Panagides J. The 4-Item Negative Symptom Assessment (NSA-4) instrument: a simple tool for evaluating negative symptoms in schizophrenia following brief training. *Psychiatry (Edgemont)*. 2010;7:26-32.

2. Depression and suicidality

Jean Addington

Depression

Depression is a common feature of schizophrenia. It is both a predictor of suicide and attempted suicide and an important correlate of quality of life. Depression is evident throughout the course of schizophrenia and is often most common at the first episode of psychosis [1,2]. In fact, young people experiencing their first episode of psychosis are at the highest risk of suicide and more often are diagnosed with depression. Thus, it was deemed important that depression should be regularly assessed in schizophrenia patients. However, one of the concerns in accurately assessing depression in schizophrenia was overlap with negative symptoms. The Calgary Depression Scale for Schizophrenia (CDSS) was developed to avoid this overlap and to have a scale that was valid for those who have schizophrenia [3]. The CDSS was shown to be both valid and reliable [4] and specific for depression in schizophrenia (ie, the degree to which it measures depression and not negative symptoms) [5]. In comparison to other scales of depression not specifically developed for schizophrenia, the CDSS did not overlap with either the positive or negative symptoms of schizophrenia [6]. Thus, the CDSS is a valid measure of depression with high internal and inter-rater reliability, all items are predictive of major depression, and it is specific to depression in schizophrenia. The CDSS has been translated into over 30 languages [7] and is used worldwide.

Using the Calgary Depression Scale for Schizophrenia

The CDSS is a nine-item instrument that is rated on a 4-point scale, 0–3 (Figure 2.1) [3]. The scale is designed to reflect the presence of depression exclusive of other dimensions of psychopathology in schizophrenia at both the acute and residual stages of the disorder. It is sensitive to change and can be used at a variety of intervals. The rater should have experience with people with schizophrenia and should develop inter-rater reliability with another rater experienced in the use of structured assessment instruments. The first question for each item should be asked as written. Follow-up probes or qualifiers are then used at the rater's discretion. The time frame refers to the previous 2 weeks unless stipulated. The last item, item 9, is based on observations during the entire interview.

R. Keefe (ed.), *Guide to Assessment Scales in Schizophrenia*,
DOI: 10.1007/978-1-908517-71-5_2,
© Springer Healthcare, a part of Springer Science+Business Media 2012

Figure 2.1 The Calgary Depression Scale for Schizophrenia

Interviewer: Ask the first question as written. Use follow up probes or qualifiers at your discretion. Time frame refers to previous 2 weeks unless stipulated. Item 9 is based on observations of the entire interview.

1. Depression: How would you describe your mood over the last 2 weeks? Do you keep reasonably cheerful or have you been very depressed or low spirited recently? In the last 2 weeks how often have you (own words) every day? All day?

0 = Absent

1 = Mild
Expresses some sadness or discouragement on questioning.

2 = Moderate
Distinct depressed mood persisting up to half the time over 2 weeks: present daily.

3 = Severe
Markedly depressed mood persisting daily over half the time interfering with normal motor and social functioning.

2. Hopelessness: How do you see the future for yourself? Can you see any future? – or has life seemed quite hopeless? Have you given up or does there still seem some reason for trying?

0 = Absent

1 = Mild
Has at times felt hopeless over the previous 2 weeks but still has some degree of hope for the future.

2 = Moderate
Persistent, moderate sense of hopelessness over last week. Can be persuaded to acknowledge possibility of things being better.

3 = Severe
Persisting and distressing sense of hopelessness.

3. Self-depreciation: What is your opinion of your self compared to other people? Do you feel better, not as good, or about the same as others? Do you feel inferior or even worthless?

0 = Absent

1 = Mild
Some inferiority; not amounting to feeling of worthlessness.

2 = Moderate
Subject feels worthless, but less than 50% of the time.

3 = Severe
Subject feels worthless more than 50% of the time. May be challenged to acknowledge otherwise.

4. Guilty ideas of reference: Do you have the feeling that you are being blamed for something or even wrongly accused? What about? (Do not include justifiable blame or accusation. Exclude delusions of guilt.)

0 = Absent

1 = Mild
Subject feels blamed but not accused less than 50% of the time.

2 = Moderate
Persisting sense of being blamed, and/or occasional sense of being accused.

3 = Severe
Persistent sense of being accused. When challenged, acknowledges that it is not so.

(continues opposite).

Figure 2.1 The Calgary Depression Scale for Schizophrenia (continued)

5. Pathological guilt: Do you tend to blame yourself for little things you may have done in the past? Do you think that you deserve to be so concerned about this?

0 = Absent

1 = Mild
Subject sometimes feels over guilty about some minor peccadillo, but less than 50% of time.

2 = Moderate
Subject usually (over 50% of time) feels guilty about past actions, the significance of which she/he exaggerates.

3 = Severe
Subject usually feels she/he is to blame for everything that has gone wrong, even when not his/her fault.

6. Morning depression: When you have felt depressed over the last 2 weeks have you noticed the depression being worse at any particular time of day?

0 = Absent
No depression.

1 = Mild
Depression present but no diurnal variation.

2 = Moderate
Depression spontaneously mentioned to be worse in the morning.

3 = Severe
Depression markedly worse in the morning, with impaired functioning that improves in the afternoon/evening.

7. Early wakening: Do you wake earlier in the morning than is normal for you? How many times a week does this happen?

0 = Absent
No early wakening.

1 = Mild
Occasionally wakes (up to twice weekly) 1 hour or more before normal time to wake or alarm time.

2 = Moderate
Often wakes early (up to 5 times weekly) 1 hour or more before normal time to wake or alarm time.

3 = Severe
Daily wakes 1 hour or more before normal time.

8. Suicide: Have you felt that life wasn't worth living? Did you ever feel like ending it all? What did you think you might do? Did you actually try?

0 = Absent

1 = Mild
Frequent thoughts of being better off dead or occasional thoughts of suicide.

2 = Moderate
Deliberately considered suicide with a plan but made no attempt.

3 = Severe
Suicidal attempt apparently designed to end in death (ie, accidental discovery or inefficient means).

(continues overleaf).

Figure 2.1 The Calgary Depression Scale for Schizophrenia (continued)

9. Observed depression: Based on interviewer's observations during the entire interview. The question "Do you feel like crying?," used at appropriate points in the interview, may elicit information useful to this observation

0 = Absent

1 = Mild
Subject appears sad and mournful, even during parts of the interview involving affectively neutral discussion.

2 = Moderate
Subject appears sad and mournful throughout the interview, with gloomy monotonous voice, and is tearful or close to tears at times.

3 = Severe
Subject chokes on distressing topics, frequently sighs deeply and cries openly, or is persistently in a state of frozen misery if examiner is sure that this is present.

(continued). Data from Addington et al [3]. © 2003, reproduced with permission from Elsevier.

Suicidality

Despite the fact that suicide is more common in individuals with schizophrenia than in the general population, there are no clear guidelines as to what are reliable risk factors for suicidality in those with schizophrenia [8]. This may account for the lack of assessment tools specifically designed to assess suicidality in those individuals with schizophrenia. The majority of rating scales used to assess suicidality typically are based on patients with other diagnoses [8].

The one specifically designed scale is the International Suicide Prevention Trial (InterSePT) Scale for Suicidal Thinking (ISST). This scale was developed for the InterSePT trial [9,10]. The ISST demonstrated robust psychometric properties such as good inter-rater reliability, and internal reliability. The ISST was compared to the CDSS to determine their effectiveness in predicting suicide attempts or hospitalizations to prevent suicide attempts [10]. Those who experienced such an event did have significant worsening on the scales between the two time points leading up to the event. Importantly, both the ISST and the CDSS were neither sensitive nor specific enough to provide a definite warning of a suicide attempt or a hospitalization to prevent an attempt. They did, however, provide some additional warnings, including, for example, overall higher ratings, slower improvement in suicidality once treatment commenced, and previous number of suicide attempts [10]. At best, the scales offer some additional information that can assist clinical decision-making regarding suicidal risk in patients with schizophrenia. Thus, the ISST may be useful to offer some clinical insights into suicidal thinking in schizophrenia patients but it is not adequate on its own to reliably detect an imminent suicidal event [10].

Using the InterSePT Scale for Suicidal Thinking
The ISST is a short scale with 12 clinically based questions that facilitate its administration. The patients should be rated based on the highest rating in the last 7 days (Figure 2.2) [9].

Figure 2.2 The InterSePT Scale for Suicidal Thinking

Rate the patient based on the highest rating in the last 7 days				Score
1. Wish to die	0 = None	1 = Weak	2 = Moderate to strong	
2. Reasons for living versus dying	0 = For living outweigh for dying	1 = About equal	2 = For dying outweigh for living	
3. Desire to make active suicide attempt	0 = None	1 = Weak	2 = Moderate to strong	
4. Passive suicidal desire	0 = Would take precautions to save life	1 = Would leave life/death to chance	2 = Would avoid steps necessary to save or maintain life	
5. Frequency of suicidal ideation	0 = Rare or occasional	1 = Intermittent	2 = Persistent or continuous	
6. Attitude toward ideation/wish	0 = Rejecting	1 = Ambivalent or indifferent	2 = Accepting	
7. Control over suicidal action/acting out/or delusions/ hallucinations of self-harm	0 = Has complete ability to control impulses	1 = Unsure of ability to control impulses	2 = Has no ability to control impulses	
8. Deterrents to active attempt (eg, religious values, family)	0 = Would not attempt because of deterrents	1 = Some concerns about deterrents	2 = Minimal or no deterrents	
9. Reason for contemplating attempt	0 = To manipulate the environment; revenge; get attention	1 = Combination of 0 and 2	2 = Escape, solve problems, psychotic reasons	
10. Method: specificity/ planning of contemplated attempt	0 = Not considered or not applicable	1 = Considered, but details not worked out	2 = Details worked out; well-formulated plan	
11. Expectancy/ anticipation by patient of actual attempt	0 = None	1 = Uncertain	2 = Yes	
12. Delusions/ hallucinations of self-harm (including command hallucinations)	0 = None	1 = Occasional	2 = Frequent	

Data from Lindenmayer et al [9]. © 1990, reproduced with permission from Elsevier.

References

1 Addington D, Addington J, Patten S. Depression in people with first-episode schizophrenia. *Br J Psychiatry.* 1998;172:90-92.

2 Addington J, Leriger E, Addington D. Symptom outcome one year after admission to an early psychosis program. *Can J Psychiatry.* 2003;48:204-207.

3 Addington D, Addington J, Schissel B. A depression rating scale for schizophrenics. *Schizophr Res.* 1990;3:247-251.

4 Addington D, Addington J, Maticka-Tyndale E, Joyce J. Reliability and validity of a depression rating scale for schizophrenics. *Schizophr Res.* 1992;6:201-208.

5 Addington D, Addington J, Maticka-Tyndale E. Specificity of the Calgary Depression Scale for schizophrenics. *Schizophr Res.* 1994;11:239-244.

6 Addington D, Addington J, Atkinson M. A psychometric comparison of the Calgary Depression Scale for Schizophrenia and the Hamilton Depression Rating Scale. *Schizophr Res.* 1996;19:205-212.

7 Addington D, Addington J. The Calgary Depression Scale for Schizophrenia. Available at: www.ucalgary.ca/cdss. Accessed April 2, 2012.

8 Preston E, Hansen L. A systematic review of suicide rating scales in schizophrenia. *Crisis.* 2005;26:170-180.

9 Lindenmayer JP, Czobor P, Alphs L, et al. The InterSePT scale for suicidal thinking reliability and validity. *Schizophr Res.* 2003;63:161-170.

10 Ayer DW, Jayathilake K, Meltzer HY. The InterSePT suicide scale for prediction of imminent suicidal behaviors. *Psychiatry Res.* 2008;161:87-96.

3. Cognition

Michael Kraus and Richard Keefe

Neurocognitive deficits are a core component of schizophrenia, with moderately severe to severe impairments seen across multiple domains of cognition on average [1,2]. Cognitive impairment is pervasive; nearly all individuals with schizophrenia present with cognitive performance below that expected if they had not developed the disease [3]. Unlike positive symptoms, cognitive deficits correlate highly with measures of functional outcome, both cross-sectionally and longitudinally [4,5]. Spurred by the pervasiveness, severity and relevance of cognitive deficits in schizophrenia, the Diagnostic and Statistical Manual of Mental Disorders (DSM-V) working group is considering including a formal cognitive criterion to the next edition of the DSM [6].

Due to the growing appreciation of the central importance of cognitive impairments in schizophrenia, tools to assess cognition in schizophrenia are of great importance. The instruments typically used to measure cognitive function in schizophrenia fall into three main categories:

1. Performance-based assessment batteries comprised of standard (mostly paper–pencil based) neuropsychological tests.
2. Computerized performance-based test batteries.
3. Interview-based assessments.

The instruments vary widely in their required testing time. A thorough neuropsychological assessment can require several hours of assessment time and enables a full evaluation of cognitive strengths and weaknesses across a broad range of neuropsychological domains. Such an assessment is usually completed or supervised by a licensed psychologist. The batteries described here are relatively brief. They capture much of the variance in overall cognition as measured by the composite score of more comprehensive batteries. The list of instruments described below is not exhaustive but represents the most commonly used tools for measuring cognition in schizophrenia. Since many psychological assessments have copyright restrictions, they are not reproduced here. Information on how to obtain them is provided.

Useful resources for clinicians to use are:

- the Wechsler Adult Intelligence Scale (WAIS) [7];
- the Wechsler Memory Scale (WMS) [8];
- the Measurement and Treatment Research to Improve Cognition in Schizophrenia (MATRICS) cognitive test [9];

R. Keefe (ed.), *Guide to Assessment Scales in Schizophrenia*,
DOI: 10.1007/978-1-908517-71-5_3,
© Springer Healthcare, a part of Springer Science+Business Media 2012

- the Repeatable Battery for the Assessment of Neuropsychological Status (RBANS) [10];
- the Brief Assessment of Cognition in Schizophrenia (BACS) [11];
- the Cambridge Neuropsychological Test Automated Battery (CANTAB) schizophrenia assessment [12];
- the CogState Schizophrenia Battery [13]; and
- the computerized cognitive testing Cognitive Drug Research (CDR) system [14].

Paper–pencil batteries

Standard neuropsychological test batteries offer several advantages. The psychometric properties of the tests are generally well established and normative data are available in many cases. The interpersonal interaction that is fundamental to the administration of these batteries allows greater flexibility in testing people with schizophrenia, and may feel less intimidating to some patients than the computer-based batteries. The pencil–paper testing process generally results in a higher completion rate than computerized tests [15]. The traditional neuropsychological tests tend to require more training than more automated computerized batteries or instruments using an interview format familiar to clinicians.

Wechsler Adult Intelligence Scale and Wechsler Memory Scale

The WAIS [7] and WMS [8] have long been the most widely employed batteries of assessment of intelligence and memory in normal populations. However, the WAIS-III alone requires approximately 100 minutes for completion in a mixed clinical population [16]. For studies of schizophrenia patient populations, researchers using these batteries have tended to reduce the number of subtests administered to reduce demands on the patients and staff. Blyler et al used regression analysis to determine the four tests covering all four domains of functioning assessed by the WAIS-III that would best account for the variance in full-scale intelligence quotient (IQ) in a sample of 41 outpatients with schizophrenia [17]. They found that a shortened version of the WAIS-III, consisting of information, block design, arithmetic, and digit symbol subtests accounted for 90% of the variance seen in the full-scale IQ of the schizophrenia patient sample and took only 30 minutes to administer [17]. Because of its brevity, the shortened version of the WAIS may have utility as a routine measure of IQ in clinical practice.

MATRICS Consensus Cognitive Battery

The US National Institutes of Health (NIH) and Food and Drug Administration (FDA) supported the MATRICS project to derive a cognitive test battery that could be used to measure treatment effects consistently across clinical studies. The result of this effort was the MATRICS Consensus Cognitive Battery (MCCB) [9,18]. From the more than 90 tests nominated for inclusion, a final battery of ten tests was chosen with an eye toward practicality of administration, favorable psychometric characteristics, demonstrated relationship to functional outcome, and adequate coverage of the domains identified as important through the MATRICS process. The MCCB requires 65 minutes to administer and allows for measurement of cognition in seven different cognitive domains. The MCCB comes with a computerized scoring system that produces T-scores and percentiles for individual tests, cognitive domains and composite scores, corrected for age and gender based on a 300-subject normative group.

Repeatable Battery for the Assessment of Neuropsychological Status

The RBANS is a brief assessment (45 minutes) originally designed to test cognitive performance in elderly patients. It has shown utility in providing reliable assessment of cognitive performance in schizophrenia patient populations [10,19,20]. The performance of patients with schizophrenia on the RBANS has been shown to be highly correlated with performance on the much longer WAIS-III and WMS-III batteries [21,22]. Because it was designed to be administered repeatedly, the RBANS does not suffer from large practice effects. However, because the battery was developed to test for dementia, it is composed largely of tests of memory, language, and visual perception and may suffer from ceiling effects on some subtests when used in a schizophrenia patient population. Also, the battery lacks measures of motor, executive and working memory performance, cognitive domains thought to be important in the cognitive impairment observed in schizophrenia. Despite these omissions, the RBANS is an appealing tool for assessment of cognition in routine clinical practice due to its relative brevity.

Brief Assessment of Cognition in Schizophrenia

The BACS battery retains the positive attributes of the RBANS (brevity of administration and scoring, repeatability, and portability) while more completely assessing the extent of cognitive impairment over multiple domains thought to be effected by schizophrenia (executive functions, verbal fluency, attention, verbal memory, working memory, and motor speed) [11]. The BACS is available in over 30 languages, has alternate forms to minimize practice effects, requires approximately 30 minutes to complete and is devised for easy administration and scoring. A spreadsheet is available for generation of composite scores by comparison to a normative sample of 400 healthy controls. The sensitivity, reliability, validity, and comparability of BACS forms have been established empirically [23]. The BACS also has clear functional relevance as the composite score is strongly related to functional measures such as independent living skills (r=0.45) and performance-based assessment of functioning (r=0.56) [24]. The BACS is well suited to routine clinical administration in which a quick assessment of overall cognitive functioning is required. Computerized and tablet versions of the BACS are available but, as of the date of this publication, have not yet been fully validated.

Brief Cognitive Assessment and Brief Cognitive Assessment Tool for Schizophrenia

Two very short batteries are the Brief Cognitive Assessment (BCA) and the Brief Cognitive Assessment Tool for Schizophrenia (B-CATS). These batteries are compositions of existing tests that were designed to assess cognition in schizophrenia patients in 15 minutes. They have good test–retest reliability, strong correlations with larger batteries, and good correlations with measures of functional ability [25,26]. The extreme brevity of the BCA and the B-CATS allow their use in routine clinical administration. The challenge for clinicians is that the tests that comprise these batteries need to be purchased separately from psychological assessment companies such as PAR, Inc. and the Psychological Corporation.

Computerized batteries

A recent development in cognitive assessment for clinical trials is the availability of computerized test batteries that allow direct data transfer to study databases. These methods minimize rater error and reduce the costs required for human quality assurance. However, some training is required. In addition, the high rate of invalid data in the assessment of people with schizophrenia compared to standardized test procedures has slowed their popularity among some clinicians and researchers.

Cambridge Neuropsychological Test Automated Battery

The CANTAB schizophrenia battery is composed of eight tests covering all seven of the MATRICS domains and requires 70 minutes of assessment time [12]. The CANTAB is presented on a touch screen computer and the nonverbal nature of most of the tests makes it an ideal battery for use in multilingual contexts. The neural bases of the CANTAB tests have been well established in animal models and human imaging studies thus allowing interpretation of results to be informed by this vast literature. The test–retest reliabilities of select CANTAB tests mostly appear promising [27].

CogState

The CogState schizophrenia battery is composed of eight tests covering all seven of the domains of cognition recommended by the MATRICS initiative [13]. Composite scores for the CogState schizophrenia battery correlate strongly with MCCB composite scores in schizophrenia subjects (r=0.83), while correlations between CogState and MCCB domain scores ranged from moderate to strong [28]. The battery requires approximately 35 minutes to complete and is suitable for testing in most countries due to the use of culture-neutral stimuli.

Cognitive Drug Research

The CDR battery was designed for repeated testing in clinical trials and has been used to study effects of disease and treatment on cognition in a variety of conditions, including schizophrenia [14]. The standard CDR can be completed in approximately 20 minutes and assesses the domains of power of attention, continuity of attention, working memory, episodic memory, and speed of memory. Individual tests can be removed from or added to the battery, which relies heavily on timed testing. The CDR has been translated into close to 60 languages and has more than 70 parallel forms.

Interview-based assessments

Interview-based assessments offer a relatively quick measure of cognition using a rating scale that may be more familiar to clinicians without a formal assessment background. Because these tools pose questions about common cognitive experiences, they are considered more face valid than standard cognitive test batteries. Step-wise regression analysis indicates that both of the interview-based assessments described below account for significant variance in real-world functioning beyond that explained by standard cognitive test batteries and measures of functional capacity, and thus may tap into aspects of cognition not fully overlapping those assessed by standard cognitive test batteries [29,30].

Schizophrenia Cognition Rating Scale

The Schizophrenia Cognition Rating Scale (SCoRS) is a 20-item interview-based assessment covering all cognitive domains tested in the MATRICS battery, and takes approximately 12 minutes to complete [29]. It is administered separately to the patient and to an informant (family, friend, social worker, etc). The interviewer is asked to rate the patient's level of difficulty performing various cognitive functions on a 4-point scale, with 4 being the most difficult and 1 being the least difficult (Figure 3.1) [29]. Upon completion of the 20 items, the interviewee is asked to give a global rating of the patient's cognitive functioning on a scale of 1 to 10. After the interview is administered to both the patient and the informant, the interviewer ranks the patient on all 20 items, and gives a global score, based on the responses of both the patient and informant as well as the interviewer's observations of the patient. The interview is available in several languages.

Empirical evaluations of the SCoRS have demonstrated high inter-rater reliability and significant correlations with measures of performance-based cognition (such as BACS), performance-based assessment of function and real-world assessment of function. Because patient scores have been found to account for little variance in cognitive performance, functional capacity or real-world functioning scores beyond that accounted for by informant ratings [29], it is possible that informant ratings alone could be collected in cases when an informant has sufficient contact with the patient.

Cognitive Assessment Interview

The Cognitive Assessment Interview (CAI) contains ten items selected from a longer interview-based assessment, the Clinical Global Impression of Cognition in Schizophrenia (CGI-CogS), by means of classical test theory and item-response theory [30]. The CAI items cover six of the seven MATRICS domains and are administered to both patients and informants and subsequently rated by the interviewer (Figure 3.2). Each of the ten individual items are rated on a seven point scale, referenced to healthy individuals of similar educational and sociocultural backgrounds. Summary ratings include global severity of cognitive impairment as judged from the patient interview, informant interview and a composite of both interviews (all rated on a seven point scale) as well as global rating of cognitive

Figure 3.1 Baseline form – Schizophrenia Cognition Rating Scale

Patient initials:	Patient randomization number:
Date of patient interview:	Date of informant interview:
Informant's relationship to patient:	Number of hours spent with patient per week:

The purpose of this questionnaire is to assess problems in attention, memory, motor skills, speech, and problem solving. The questions are designed to measure the patient's severity of cognitive difficulty within the past 2 weeks. There are a total of 20 questions to be asked of the patient and then the informant in separate interviews. As the interviewer, you will determine your rating based upon your interviews of both the patient and the informant. Please circle the appropriate whole number for each question.

Level of severity:	N/A = Rating not applicable	1 = None	2 = Mild	3 = Moderate	4 = Severe

Do you/does the patient have difficulty...

1. Remembering names of people you know or meet? (eg, roommate, nurse, doctor, family and friends)

Mild: Remembers most names of people that he/she knows but not all of the people he/she has just met.

Moderate: Forgets many names of people he/she knows and all of the names of people he/she has just met.

Severe: Forgets all or almost all names of people he/she knows and meets.

Patient					Informant					Interviewer				
N/A	1	2	3	4	N/A	1	2	3	4	N/A	1	2	3	4

2. Remembering how to get places? (eg, restroom, own room, friend's house)

Mild: Forgets infrequently.

Moderate: Is only able to get to frequently visited places.

Severe: Unable to get anyplace without assistance because difficulties with memory.

Patient					Informant					Interviewer				
N/A	1	2	3	4	N/A	1	2	3	4	N/A	1	2	3	4

3. Following/understanding a TV show? (eg, favorite show, news)

Mild: Can only follow a short movie or news show.

Moderate: Can only follow a light, 30-minute show (ie, sitcom).

Severe: Unable to follow a TV show for any period of time.

Patient					Informant					Interviewer				
N/A	1	2	3	4	N/A	1	2	3	4	N/A	1	2	3	4

4. Remembering where you put things? (eg, clothes, newspaper, cigarettes)

Mild: Rare instances of forgetfulness.

Moderate: Frequent instances of forgetfulness.

Severe: Very frequent instances of forgetfulness or forgetting items of great importance.

Patient					Informant					Interviewer				
N/A	1	2	3	4	N/A	1	2	3	4	N/A	1	2	3	4

(continues opposite).

Figure 3.1 Baseline form – Schizophrenia Cognition Rating Scale (continued)

5. Remembering your chores and responsibilities? (eg, household chores, appointments)

Mild: Infrequently forgets.

Moderate: Forgets only those things that do not occur everyday.

Severe: Forgets all or almost all of his/her responsibilities.

Patient					Informant					Interviewer				
N/A	1	2	3	4	N/A	1	2	3	4	N/A	1	2	3	4

6. Learning how to use new gadgets and equipment? (eg, computers, washer, microwave, phone, remote, TV)

Mild: Takes longer to learn than most, but can usually do it.

Moderate: Takes longer and needs to be taught; cannot learn some things.

Severe: Unable to learn how to use new gadgets and equipment.

Patient					Informant					Interviewer				
N/A	1	2	3	4	N/A	1	2	3	4	N/A	1	2	3	4

7. Remembering information and/or instructions recently given to you? (eg, telephone numbers, directions, names)

Mild: Rarely has difficulty remembering information.

Moderate: Frequently forgets information given.

Severe: Almost always forgets information.

Patient					Informant					Interviewer				
N/A	1	2	3	4	N/A	1	2	3	4	N/A	1	2	3	4

8. Remembering what you were going to say? (eg, forgetting words, stopping mid-sentence)

Mild: Rare instances of forgetfulness when speaking.

Moderate: Rare instances of forgetfulness when speaking.

Severe: Frequency of forgetfulness makes communication very difficult.

Patient					Informant					Interviewer				
N/A	1	2	3	4	N/A	1	2	3	4	N/A	1	2	3	4

9. Keeping track of your money? (eg, managing bills, counting change)

Mild: Some difficulty but can usually do it.

Moderate: Significant difficulty either with counting change or paying bills.

Severe: Unable to keep track of his/her money because of cognitive difficulties.

Patient					Informant					Interviewer				
N/A	1	2	3	4	N/A	1	2	3	4	N/A	1	2	3	4

10. Keeping your words from being jumbled together? (eg, words get mixed up or 'run together')

Mild: Sometimes will jumble words but it's rare.

Moderate: Can have a conversation but jumbles words frequently.

Severe: Unable to have a conversation due to jumbled words.

Patient					Informant					Interviewer				
N/A	1	2	3	4	N/A	1	2	3	4	N/A	1	2	3	4

(continues overleaf).

Figure 3.1 Baseline form – Schizophrenia Cognition Rating Scale (continued)

11. Concentrating well enough to read a newspaper or a book? (eg, reading same sentence or page over and over)

Mild: Can concentrate except for rare occasions.
Moderate: Can concentrate on short and easy to understand materials.
Severe: Unable to read even the simplest materials due to concentration problems.

Patient					Informant					Interviewer				
N/A	1	2	3	4	N/A	1	2	3	4	N/A	1	2	3	4

12. With familiar tasks? (eg, cooking, driving, showering, getting dressed)

Mild: Rarely has difficulty completing the task.
Moderate: Frequently needs verbal assistance to complete the task.
Severe: Needs physical assistance to do these tasks due to cognitive difficulties.

Patient					Informant					Interviewer				
N/A	1	2	3	4	N/A	1	2	3	4	N/A	1	2	3	4

13. Staying focused? (eg, daydream, trouble paying attention to someone talking)

Mild: Sometimes unable to stay focused.
Moderate: Frequently unable to stay focused.
Severe: Almost always unable to stay focused.

Patient					Informant					Interviewer				
N/A	1	2	3	4	N/A	1	2	3	4	N/A	1	2	3	4

14. Learning new things? (eg, new words, new ways of doing things, new schedules)

Mild: Takes longer to learn than most, but can usually do it.
Moderate: Takes longer and needs special attention.
Severe: Unable to learn almost all new things.

Patient					Informant					Interviewer				
N/A	1	2	3	4	N/A	1	2	3	4	N/A	1	2	3	4

15. Speaking as fast as you would like? (eg, slow speech, pauses)

Mild: Rarely speaks slowly because of cognitive difficulties.
Moderate: Often speaks slowly because of cognitive difficulties.
Severe: Ability to converse is jeopardized because of cognitive difficulties.

Patient					Informant					Interviewer				
N/A	1	2	3	4	N/A	1	2	3	4	N/A	1	2	3	4

16. Doing things quickly? (eg, writing, lighting a cigarette)

Mild: Slightly slower than normal pace.
Moderate: Significantly slower; may need prompting to do things quickly.
Severe: Unable to get things done because time runs out.

Patient					Informant					Interviewer				
N/A	1	2	3	4	N/A	1	2	3	4	N/A	1	2	3	4

(continues opposite).

Figure 3.1 Baseline form – Schizophrenia Cognition Rating Scale (continued)

17. Handling changes in your daily routine? (eg, appointments, special visits, group therapy)

Mild: Can adjust with considerable effort.

Moderate: Will eventually adjust with assistance.

Severe: Changes in the daily routine are impossible.

Patient					Informant					Interviewer				
N/A	1	2	3	4	N/A	1	2	3	4	N/A	1	2	3	4

18. Understanding what people mean when they are talking to you? (eg, feeling confused by what someone says)

Mild: Some difficulty understanding what people mean.

Moderate: Often has difficulty understanding what people mean.

Severe: Frequently unable to understand what people mean.

Patient					Informant					Interviewer				
N/A	1	2	3	4	N/A	1	2	3	4	N/A	1	2	3	4

19. Understanding how other people feel about things? (eg, misunderstanding people's emotions by their facial expressions or tone of their voice)

Mild: Rarely has difficulty understanding how people feel.

Moderate: Often has difficulty understanding how people feel.

Severe: Very frequent instances of difficulty understanding how people feel.

Patient					Informant					Interviewer				
N/A	1	2	3	4	N/A	1	2	3	4	N/A	1	2	3	4

20. Following conversations in a group? (eg, participation, able to follow conversation)

Mild: Few difficulties following conversations in a group.

Moderate: Often unable to follow conversations in a group.

Severe: Frequently unable to follow conversations in a group and communication in that setting is difficult or impossible.

Patient					Informant					Interviewer				
N/A	1	2	3	4	N/A	1	2	3	4	N/A	1	2	3	4

Global rating – interviewer only

What is your overall impression of the patient's level of difficulty in these areas? (Interviewer should circle appropriate number or mark.)

(none)	1	2	3	4	5	6	7	8	9	10	(extreme)

(continued). Data from Keefe et al [29]. Reproduced with permission from Dr R Keefe. © 2001, Duke University.

Figure 3.2 Cognitive Assessment Interview

Date:	Patient ID:	
Rater:	Session:	
Background information section		
Patient domains		
Observation/evaluation	**Patient**	
Appearance – general cleanliness and hygiene, clothing (correctness of clothing for season, neatness, matching colors/prints, fasteners done)	Make notes:	
Use all sources of information	Record sources:	
Compliance		
Takes medications at correct doses and at correct times as prescribed?		
Medication changes		
General orientation		
Time (day, year, date), place (city, state, clinic), person		
Describe patient's living situation		
Is patient experiencing psychotic symptoms? (eg, hallucinations)	Please describe:	
Handedness (hand used for writing)		
Ask patient to describe relationship to informant (eg, mother, case worker) and number of contact hours per week	Record information:	
Patient and informant domains		
Relevant history	**Patient**	**Informant**
Recent relevant clinical events, illnesses of the patient, the informant or other family members, significant social or personal events. Major fluctuations in clinical state. (For follow-up exam: clinical events since baseline interview)		
Demographics		
Education level (years; HS = 12):		
Occupation/student status:		
Date of birth:		
Duration of interview:	Record in minutes:	Record in minutes:
Record notes:		

(continues opposite).

Figure 3.2 Cognitive Assessment Interview (continued)

Working memory

Severity anchor points for sections 1–4

N/A = Rating not applicable, or insufficient information.

1 = Normal, not at all impaired.

2 = Minimal cognitive deficits but functioning is generally effective.

3 = Mild cognitive deficits with some consistent effect on functioning.

4 = Moderate cognitive deficits with clear effects on functioning.

5 = Serious cognitive deficits that interfere with day-to-day functioning.

6 = Severe cognitive deficits that jeopardize independent living.

7 = Cognitive deficits are so severe as to present danger to self/others.

1. Difficulty maintaining newly learned verbal information in mind for brief periods (long enough to use)?

Do you forget names of people you just met?

Do you have trouble recalling telephone numbers you hear?

Do you have trouble remembering what your doctor just said during visits?

Do you find you need to write down information to remember?

Patient examples: Informant examples:

Patient								Informant								Composite							
N/A	1	2	3	4	5	6	7	N/A	1	2	3	4	5	6	7	N/A	1	2	3	4	5	6	7

2. Difficulty performing 'on the spot' mental manipulations or computations?

Do you have difficulty knowing how much change to expect when shopping?

Do you have trouble keeping figures in mind while paying bills or balancing your checkbook?

Patient examples: Informant examples:

Patient								Informant								Composite							
N/A	1	2	3	4	5	6	7	N/A	1	2	3	4	5	6	7	N/A	1	2	3	4	5	6	7

Attention/vigilance

3. Problems sustaining concentration over time (without distraction)?

Do you have trouble concentrating?

Do you take breaks frequently?

Do you have trouble paying attention while reading, listening to the radio or watching television, long enough to read/listen/see a whole article/chapter/program?

Patient examples: Informant examples:

Patient								Informant								Composite							
N/A	1	2	3	4	5	6	7	N/A	1	2	3	4	5	6	7	N/A	1	2	3	4	5	6	7

(continues overleaf).

Figure 3.2 Cognitive Assessment Interview (continued)

4. Difficulty focusing on select information (if there is not obvious distraction)?

Do you have trouble finding what you need at the supermarket?

Is it difficult for you to pick out the correct route on a bus map?

Patient examples:								Informant examples:														
Patient								Informant									Composite						
N/A	1	2	3	4	5	6	7	N/A	1	2	3	4	5	6	7	N/A	1	2	3	4	5	6	7

Verbal learning and memory

Severity anchor points for sections 5–9

N/A = Rating not applicable, or insufficient information.

1 = Normal, not at all impaired.

2 = Minimal cognitive deficits but functioning is generally effective.

3 = Mild cognitive deficits with some consistent effect on functioning.

4 = Moderate cognitive deficits with clear effects on functioning.

5 = Serious cognitive deficits that interfere with day-to-day functioning.

6 = Severe cognitive deficits that jeopardize independent living.

7 = Cognitive deficits are so severe as to present danger to self/others.

5. Trouble learning and remembering verbal material?

Do you have trouble learning and remembering instructions or other important information (eg, names of medications)?

Do you have trouble learning and remembering later the names of people you meet?

Do you need to have things written down to remember?

Patient examples:								Informant examples:														
Patient								Informant									Composite						
N/A	1	2	3	4	5	6	7	N/A	1	2	3	4	5	6	7	N/A	1	2	3	4	5	6	7

6. Difficulty recalling recent events?

Do you find you have to be reminded by others of events that occurred?

Do you recall what you had for dinner last night?

What's been in the news lately?

Patient examples:								Informant examples:														
Patient								Informant									Composite						
N/A	1	2	3	4	5	6	7	N/A	1	2	3	4	5	6	7	N/A	1	2	3	4	5	6	7

Reasoning and problem-solving

7. Lack of flexibility in generating alternate plans when needed?

Do you have trouble coming up with alternatives when your plans are disturbed (eg, what if your normal mode of transport was not available, or the store you usually go to was closed)?

Patient examples:								Informant examples:														
Patient								Informant									Composite						
N/A	1	2	3	4	5	6	7	N/A	1	2	3	4	5	6	7	N/A	1	2	3	4	5	6	7

(continues opposite).

Figure 3.2 Cognitive Assessment Interview (continued)

8. Problems in situations requiring judgment?

What would you do if … [your power went out/you were locked out of your home/your only sink was clogged/a light bulb went out]?

Patient examples: Informant examples:

Patient								Informant								Composite							
N/A	1	2	3	4	5	6	7	N/A	1	2	3	4	5	6	7	N/A	1	2	3	4	5	6	7

Speed of processing

9. Performs tasks slowly?

Do you find things take you longer than they should (eg, performing tasks such as cooking or shopping, assembling materials, reading instructions)?

Patient examples: Informant examples:

Patient								Informant								Composite							
N/A	1	2	3	4	5	6	7	N/A	1	2	3	4	5	6	7	N/A	1	2	3	4	5	6	7

Social cognition

Severity anchor points for section 10

N/A = Rating not applicable, or insufficient information.

1 = Normal, not at all impaired.

2 = Minimal cognitive deficits but functioning is generally effective.

3 = Mild cognitive deficits with some consistent effect on functioning.

4 = Moderate cognitive deficits with clear effects on functioning.

5 = Serious cognitive deficits that interfere with day-to-day functioning.

6 = Severe cognitive deficits that jeopardize independent living.

7 = Cognitive deficits are so severe as to present danger to self/others.

10. Difficulty appreciating another person's intentions/point of view?

Do you have trouble understanding other people's point of view (if you disagree with them; even if they don't say it outwardly)?

If you are talking and someone looks at their watch, what do you think they may be feeling?

Patient examples: Informant examples:

Patient								Informant								Composite							
N/A	1	2	3	4	5	6	7	N/A	1	2	3	4	5	6	7	N/A	1	2	3	4	5	6	7

(continues overleaf).

Figure 3.2 Cognitive Assessment Interview (continued)

Clinical global impression of cognitive impairment

Considering all sources of information gathered for this patient as compared to a community comparison sample on how the domains of neurocognitive functioning influence daily living, rate global severity of cognitive impairment, how cognitively impaired is this person? (Circle one)

Global severity of cognitive impairment – from patient interview

N/A = Not assessed	Notes:
1 = Normal, no cognitive impairment	
2 = Borderline impairment	
3 = Mildly impaired	
4 = Moderately impaired	
5 = Markedly impaired	
6 = Severely impaired	
7 = Among the most extremely impaired	

Global severity of cognitive impairment – from informant interview

N/A = Not assessed	Notes:
1 = Normal, no cognitive impairment	
2 = Borderline impairment	
3 = Mildly impaired	
4 = Moderately impaired	
5 = Markedly impaired	
6 = Severely impaired	
7 = Among the most extremely impaired	

Global severity of cognitive impairment – rater composite impression

N/A = Not assessed	Notes:
1 = Normal, no cognitive impairment	
2 = Borderline impairment	
3 = Mildly impaired	
4 = Moderately impaired	
5 = Markedly impaired	
6 = Severely impaired	
7 = Among the most extremely impaired	

(continues opposite).

Figure 3.2 Cognitive Assessment Interview (continued)

Global assessment of function – cognition in schizophrenia

91–100	Superior cognitive functioning in a wide range of activities, is sought out to work on cognitively demanding problems, maintains superior level of functioning in a cognitively demanding vocation.
81–90	Absent or minimal cognitive deficits (eg, occasional lapses of memory or word-finding difficulty), good functioning in all cognitive areas, effective functioning and engagement in cognitive tasks, no more than everyday concerns about cognitive performance.
71–80	If cognitive deficits are present, they are transient and expectable reactions to stressors (eg, difficulty concentrating after family argument), no more than slight impairment in social, occupational or school functioning due to cognitive deficits.
61–70	Some mild cognitive symptoms (eg, difficulty concentrating or memory lapses) **or** some difficulty in social, occupational or school functioning due to cognitive problems (eg, had to repeat a course in college due to cognitive problems).
51–60	Moderate cognitive symptoms (eg, persistent problems paying attention or forgetting of scheduled events) **or** moderate difficulty in social, occupational or school functioning due to cognitive problems (eg, had to take a leave of absence from school).
41–50	Serious cognitive problems (eg, continuous problems with attention, memory, or planning) **or** any serious impairment in social, occupational or school functioning due to cognitive problems (eg, family problems caused by deficits, unable to keep a job).
31–40	Severe cognitive problems interfering with multiple social, occupational, or school functions (eg, an individual is unable to work in competitive employment, has difficulty in supported employment, and has difficulty assisting with chores at residence).
21–30	Cognitive deficits are so pronounced that they interfere with virtually all aspects of functioning, including meaningful communication and goal-directed activity (eg, difficulty sustaining conversation, performing basic activities of daily living).
11–20	Some danger of harm to self or others due to cognitive deficits (gross impairments of planning/judgment, failure to recognize consequences of actions, frequently disoriented, wandering, or confused).
1–10	Persistent danger of harm to self or others **or** inability to maintain personal hygiene due to cognitive deficits (eg, no meaningful communication, inability to perform even basic self care due to problems organizing behavior).
0	Inadequate information.

Global assessment of function

Session	Patient	Informant	Composite
Baseline			
Follow-up			

(continued). Data from Ventura et al [30]. Reproduced with permission from Dr J Ventura, Dr R Bilder, Dr S Reise, and Dr R Keefe.

function on a 100-point scale. When an informant is not available, the CAI may be preferred over the SCoRS since the patient-only assessment demonstrates better test–retest reliability and relation to performance-based measures of cognition [31]. Although the CAI has fewer items, the probe questions are extensive and may require more time than the SCoRS [32].

References

1   Saykin AJ, Gur RC, Gur RE, et al. Neuropsychological function in schizophrenia. Selective impairment in memory and learning. *Arch Gen Psychiatry*. 1991;48:618-624.

2   Harvey PD, Keefe RS. Cognitive impairment in schizophrenia and implications of atypical neuroleptic treatment. *CNS Spectrums*. 1997;2:1-11.

3   Keefe RS, Eesley CE, Poe MP. Defining a cognitive function decrement in schizophrenia. *Biol Psychiatry*. 2005;57:688-691.

4   Velligan DI, Mahurin RK, Diamond PL, Hazleton BC, Eckert SL, Miller AL. The functional significance of symptomatology and cognitive function in schizophrenia. *Schizophr Res*. 1997;25:21-31.

5   Green MF, Kern RS, Heaton RK. Longitudinal studies of cognition and functional outcome in schizophrenia: implications for MATRICS. *Schizophr Res*. 2004;72:41-51.

6   Keefe RSE, Fenton WS. How should DSM-V criteria for schizophrenia include cognitive impairment? *Schizophr Bull*. 2007;33:912-920.

7   Wechsler D. Wechsler Adult Intelligence Scale – fourth edition (WAIS–IV). Available at: www.pearsonassessments.com/HAIWEB/Cultures/en-us/Productdetail.htm?Pid=015-8980-808. Accessed April 2, 2012.

8   Wechsler D. Wechsler Memory Scale – fourth edition (WMS-IV). Available at: www.pearsonassessments.com/HAIWEB/Cultures/en-us/Productdetail.htm?Pid=015-8895-800&Mode=summary. Accessed April 2, 2012.

9   MATRICS Assessment Inc. MATRICS Consensus Cognitive Battery. Available at: www.matricsinc.org/MCCB.htm. Accessed April 2, 2012.

10 Randolph C. Repeatable Battery for the Assessment of Neuropsychological Status. Available at: www.rbans.com. Accessed April 2, 2012.

11 NeuroCog Trials. Licensed instruments. Available at: www.neurocogtrials.com/licensed-instruments. Accessed April 2, 2012.

12 Cambridge Cognition. CANTAB schizophrenia. Available at: www.camcog.com/cantab-schizophrenia.asp. Accessed April 2, 2012.

13 CogState Clinical Trials. Schizophrenia battery. Available at: www.cogstate.com/go/clinicaltrials/our-test-batteries/schizophrenia-battery. Accessed April 2, 2012.

14 United Biosource. Computerized cognitive testing. Available at: www.unitedbiosource.com/specialty/computerized-cognitive-testing.aspx. Accessed April 2, 2012.

15 Silverstein SM, Jaeger J, Donovan-Lepore AM, et al. A comparative study of the MATRICS and IntegNeuro cognitive assessment batteries. *J Clin Exp Neuropsychol*. 2010;32:937-952.

16 Ryan JJ, Lopez SJ, Werth TR. Administration time estimated for WAIS-III Subtests, Scales, and Short Forms in a clinical sample. *J Psychoeduc Assess*. 1998;16:315-323.

17 Blyler CR, Gold JM, Iannone VN, Buchanan RW. Short form of the WAIS-III for use with patients with schizophrenia. *Schizophr Res*. 2000;46:209-215.

18 Nuechterlein KH, Green MF. *MATRICS Consensus Cognitive Battery Manual*. Los Angeles, USA: MATRICS Assessment Inc.; 2006.

19 Weber B. RBANS has reasonable test-retest reliability in schizophrenia. *EBMH*. 2003;6:22.

20 Wilk CM, Gold JM, Bartko JJ, et al. Test-retest stability of the Repeatable Battery for the Assessment of Neuropsychological Status in schizophrenia. *Am J Psychiatry*. 2002;159:838-844.

21 Gold JM, Queern C, Iannone VN, Buchanan RW. Repeatable Battery for the Assessment of Neuropsychological Status as a screening test in schizophrenia, I: sensitivity, reliability, and validity. *Am J Psychiatry*. 1999;156:1944-1950.

22 Hobart MP, Goldberg R, Bartko JJ, Gold JM. Repeatable Battery for the Assessment of Neuropsychological Status as a screening test in schizophrenia, II: convergent/discriminant validity and diagnostic group comparisons. *Am J Psychiatry.* 1999;156:1951-1957.

23 Keefe RSE, Goldberg TE, Harvey PD, Gold JM, Poe MP, Coughenour L. The Brief Assessment of Cognition in Schizophrenia: reliability, sensitivity, and comparison with a standard neurocognitive battery. *Schizophr Res.* 2004;68:283-297.

24 Keefe RS, Poe M, Walker TM, Harvey PD. The relationship of the Brief Assessment of Cognition in Schizophrenia (BACS) to functional capacity and real-world functional outcome. *J Clin Exp Neuropsychol.* 2006;28:260-269.

25 Velligan DI, DiCocco M, Bow-Thomas CC, et al. A brief cognitive assessment for use with schizophrenia patients in community clinics. *Schizophr Res.* 2004;71:273-283.

26 Hurford IM, Marder SR, Keefe RSE, Reise SP, Bilder RM. A brief cognitive assessment tool for schizophrenia: construction of a tool for clinicians. *Schizophr Bull.* 2011;37:538-545.

27 Barnett JH, Robbins TW, Leeson VC, Sahakian BJ, Joyce EM, Blackwell AD. Assessing cognitive function in clinical trials of schizophrenia. *Neurosci Biobehav Rev.* 2010;34:1161-1177.

28 Pietrzak RH, Olver J, Norman T, Piskulic D, Maruff P, Snyder PJ. A comparison of the CogState Schizophrenia Battery and the Measurement and Treatment Research to Improve Cognition in Schizophrenia (MATRICS) Battery in assessing cognitive impairment in chronic schizophrenia. *J Clin Exp Neuropsychol.* 2009;31:848-859.

29 Keefe RS, Poe M, Walker TM, Kang JW, Harvey PD. The Schizophrenia Cognition Rating Scale: an interview-based assessment and its relationship to cognition, real-world functioning, and functional capacity. *Am J Psychiatry.* 2006;163:426-432.

30 Ventura J, Reise SP, Keefe RSE, et al. The Cognitive Assessment Interview (CAI): development and validation of an empirically derived, brief interview-based measure of cognition. *Schizophr Res.* 2010;121:24-31.

31 Green MF, Nuechterlein KH, Kern RS, et al. Functional co-primary measures for clinical trials in schizophrenia: results from the MATRICS Psychometric and Standardization Study. *Am J Psychiatry.* 2008;165:221-228.

32 Green MF, Schooler NR, Kern RS, et al. Evaluation of functionally meaningful measures for clinical trials of cognition enhancement in schizophrenia. *Am J Psychiatry.* 2011;168:400-407.

4. Functional outcomes assessment scales

Philip D Harvey

Deficits in the performance of everyday functional skills are quite common in people with schizophrenia. These include impairments in productive activities, social functioning, and independence in residence and related activities. There are multiple strategies to assess these impairments, including assessment of achievement of various functional milestones, reporting/assessing the likelihood and capability with which these acts are performed and ratings of the skills that underlie the performance of these acts. A recent development in the assessment of disability in schizophrenia has been the focus on the direct assessment of the skills that underlie functioning in the community. Referred to as 'functional capacity,' these abilities have been shown to be more proximal to everyday functioning than impairments in cognitive performance [1].

Rating scales aimed at everyday functioning have two general formats. Some of these scales examine functioning in single domains, such as social functioning or everyday activities. Other scales adopt a more hybrid approach and rate multiple elements of functioning at the same time. Some of these rating scales are designed exclusively for the self-reporting of functioning and others are used to generate clinician or other informant ratings of functioning. The likely validity of these different approaches is discussed in this chapter.

One of the major reasons to use rating scales to examine everyday functioning in schizophrenia is the low frequency of achievement of milestones such as full-time employment, marriage or a similar stable relationship, or independence in residence [2]. As these occurrences are uncommon in patients with schizophrenia, simple tallies of milestones are likely to be hampered by low frequencies of occurrence. After all, if a milestone occurs with only 10% prevalence, ratings would be 90% accurate if it was simply assumed that the events never occurred. More important, therefore, is the ability to rate sub-milestone achievements (seeking a job, moving to a supported residence from a long-stay hospital) and to examine elements of skilled acts (managing money) that may be useful for predicting future achievements.

Table 4.1 presents a list of several different everyday functioning rating scales [3–8]. These scales were selected as the best available on the basis of the Validation of Everyday Real-World Outcomes (VALERO) Expert Survey and RAND Panel performed in 2007 [9], and have been recently compared in a systematic study by the author [12]. Some information has been collected on the relative usefulness of these six best scales for use in the assessment of people with schizophrenia

R. Keefe (ed.), *Guide to Assessment Scales in Schizophrenia*,
DOI: 10.1007/978-1-908517-71-5_4,
© Springer Healthcare, a part of Springer Science+Business Media 2012

in terms of predicting scores on performance-based ability measures and for their utility across different informants. A number of the functional status rating scales also include other assessments, such as ratings of symptoms such as disruptiveness or negative symptoms. In addition to the scales listed in Table 4.1, there are two more potentially promising scales, the Schizophrenia Objective Functioning Inventory (SOFI) [10] and the Personal and Social Performance Scale (PSP) [11], that were not included in the VALERO Expert Survey because they were too new at the time.

Similarly to the everyday functioning rating scales, an expert panel has conducted a survey on the most promising functional capacity measures [16]. This research included measures of everyday living skills because performance-based measures of social abilities are quite affected by cultural factors. Table 4.2 identifies the three functional capacity measures [13–15] that were selected as the most promising by the study.

Although the validation studies clearly have some limitations, their results provide a systematic assessment of the reliability and concurrent validity of available functional capacity and everyday functioning measures. The scales that were selected as best by the two studies as well as the newer SOFI and PSP scales will be discussed in further detail in this chapter.

Table 4.1 Everyday functioning rating scales selected by the RAND expert panel

Reference	Scale	Classification
Heinrichs et al (1984) [3]	Heinrichs-Carpenter Quality of Life Scale (QLS)	Hybrid
Schneider & Struening (1983) [4]	Specific Levels of Functioning Scale (SLOF)	Hybrid
Birchwood et al (1990) [5]	Birchwood Social Functioning Scale (SFS)	Social functioning
Wykes & Stuart (1986) [6]	Social Behavior Schedule (SBS)	Social functioning
Rosen et al (1989) [7]	Life Skills Profile (LSP)	Everyday living
Wallace et al (2000) [8]	Independent Living Skills Survey (ILSS)	Everyday living

Data from Leifker et al [9].

Table 4.2 Functional capacity measures examined in Measures for Clinical Trials of Treatment of Cognitive Impairment

Reference	Scale
Patterson et al (2001) [13]	University of California, San Diego (UCSD) Performance-Based Skills Assessment (UPSA)
Velligan et al (2007) [14]	Test of Adaptive Behavior In Schizophrenia (TABS)
Loeb (1996) [15]	Independent Living Scales (ILS)

Data from Green et al [16].

Functional rating scales

Specific Levels of Functioning Scale

The Specific Levels of Functioning Scale (SLOF) is a 43-item multidimensional behavioral survey administered in person to the caseworker or caregiver of a patient with schizophrenia [4]. The scale assesses the patient's current functioning and behavior across the following six domains:

1. Physical functioning.
2. Personal care skills.
3. Interpersonal relationships.
4. Social acceptability.
5. Activities of community living.
6. Work skills.

Each of the questions in the above domains is rated on a 5-point Likert scale. Scores on the instrument range from 43 to 215. The higher the total score, the better overall functioning of the patient. The exact time frame that the survey attempts to assess functioning for is unspecified. The scale also includes an open-ended question asking the informant if there are any other areas of functioning not covered by the instrument that may be important in assessing functioning in this patient. Each informant is asked to rank how well they know the patient on a 5-point Likert scale ranging from 'not well at all' to 'very well.'

In a systematic study [12] comparing the simultaneous correlation of the six everyday functioning rating scales listed in Table 4.1 with three performance-based measures of patients abilities, the SLOF proved most highly correlated with the ability measures. The procedure used is critical, in that an interviewer saw the patient and had them complete all six rating scales and then saw an informant, who also completed the same scales. The interviewer then generated their own best-estimate judgment of the patient's 'true' level of functioning. These ratings were then used to perform complex correlation analyses, which suggested the SLOF was most highly correlated of all the scales with performance-based outcomes. These results do not indicate that other scales are not useful, only that the SLOF was rated the highest in this study.

Schizophrenia Objective Functioning Inventory

One functional rating scale that was not nominated by experts in 2007 [9], but which has been the subject of some interesting analyses over the last 4 years, is the SOFI [10]. The SOFI was developed to measure functional deficits due to patient psychopathology and cognitive impairment. The SOFI rates four domains considered most relevant to a functional outcome measure in schizophrenia:

1. Living situation (stability, structure/supervision, independence).
2. Instrumental activities of daily living (financial management, transportation, medication, treatment, housework/childcare, self-care, shopping, food/cooking, planning, and leisure activities).

3. Productive activities (work, other vocational-oriented activities, treatment-related activities, education, homemaking/childcare).
4. Social functioning (social activity and social support).

There are interviewer and patient self-report versions of the SOFI and these both have a set of probe questions that lead to scores that are scaled in a similar way to the Global Assessment of Functioning (GAF): a 0–100 scale with each ten-point interval defining an increasingly higher level of functioning, up to a maximum score of 100. The SOFI has not yet been widely used.

The Personal and Social Performance Scale

Similar to the SOFI, the PSP was also not nominated by the VALERO Expert Panel in 2007 [9]. It is a clinician-rated scale examining interpersonal and social functioning, as well as the ability to perform activities of daily living and to avoid being socially disruptive [11]. The PSP is also scored using GAF-like criteria, which generate scores that are then clinically interpreted in terms of their placement in 10-point intervals that define different levels of functional and social outcomes. A structured interview with the patient and caregiver, as well as structured observation, is used to generate the ratings, which lead to an overall score ranging from 0 to 100. Scores of 70 and above are designated as reflecting mild levels of impairment.

Everyday functioning scales

Some of the everyday functioning scales accompany structured interviews that may take an extended period to complete. Thus, these scales are difficult to employ with certain classes of informants and are not possible to administer without face-to-face contact. Other scales also have been developed to be administered as questionnaires, which have the benefit of being able to be mailed to research participants or informants. There is considerable information to suggest that patient self-reports, in the absence of information from certain types of informants, manifest very little overlap with other indices of functioning. Thus, rating everyday functioning in schizophrenia is best accomplished by utilizing multiple sources of information, including records, interviewers with informants, patient self-report, and a skillful interviewer who can then make a judgment about patients' 'true' levels of functioning. Collecting self-reports alone has repeatedly been found to generate unreliable results and should never be used as an outcome measure in a treatment study.

Functional capacity measures

The functional capacity scales described in Table 4.2 [13–15] were compared in a systematic study, the Measures for Clinical Trials of Treatment of Cognitive Impairment (MATRICS-CT) [16]. They were each examined for several critical psychometric characteristics, as well as for their ease of use and tolerability to patients. The results of the study suggested that the University of California, San Diego (UCSD) Performance- based Skills Assessment (UPSA) was the best of these scales, based on its highest correlations with cognition, it being the most efficient and tolerable measure, and general impressions of user friendliness. Each scale was examined in a long and abbreviated version.

Conclusions

The results of the comparative study indicated that the long version of the UPSA was the most suitable form and that short forms of the UPSA and Test of Adaptive Behavior in Schizophrenia (TABS) were both acceptable and quite similar. Although the UPSA was seen to be more useful than the TABS, the ratings for the TABS were quite good and some content domains in the TABS do not overlap with the UPSA. Thus, we present both the TABS and UPSA as available performance-based measures of functional capacity. It is important to emphasize that performance-based functional capacity measures are used as co-primary outcomes in cognitive enhancement trials in schizophrenia, as directed by the FDA. Understanding the mechanics of these measures is important for individuals attempting to design trials of cognitive enhancement, including both pharmacological and cognitive remediation measures.

Furthermore, in-depth study of all of the important issues associated with functional assessments, including both abilities and real-world outcomes, is recommended as they cannot be addressed in full here. Several of the papers cited, including Harvey et al [10], Green et al [16], and Leifker et al [9], have detailed descriptions of the issues associated with assessment of everyday functioning and functional capacity.

References

1 Harvey PD, Bellack AS, Velligan D. Performance-based measures of functional skills: usefulness in clinical treatment studies. *Schizophr Bull.* 2007;33:1138-1148.

2 Leung WW, Bowie CR, Harvey PD. Functional Implications of Neuropsychological Normality and Symptom Remission in Schizophrenia: a cross-sectional study. *J Int Neuropsychol Soc.* 2008;14:479-488.

3 Heinrichs DW, Hanlon TE, Carpenter WT. The Quality of Life Scale: an instrument for rating the schizophrenia deficit syndrome. *Schizophr Bull.* 1984;10:388-396.

4 Schneider LC, Struening EL. SLOF: a behavioral rating scale for assessing the mentally ill. *Soc Work Res Abstr.* 1983;19:9-21.

5 Birchwood M, Smith J, Cochrane R, Wetton S, Copestake S. The Social Functioning Scale: the development and validation of a new scale of social adjustment for use in family intervention programmes with schizophrenic patients. *Br J Psychiatry.* 1990;157:853-859.

6 Wykes T, Stuart E. The measurement of social behavior in psychiatric patients: and assessment of the reliability and validity of the SBS schedule. *Br J Psychiatry.* 1986;148:1-11.

7 Rosen A, Hadzi-Pavlovic D, Parker G. The Life Skills Profile: a measure assessing function and disability in schizophrenia. *Schizophr Bull.* 1989;15:325-337.

8 Wallace C J, Liberman RP, Tauber R, Wallace J. The Independent Living Skills Survey: a comprehensive measure of the community functioning of severely and persistently mentally ill individuals. *Schizophr Bull.* 2000;26:631-658.

9 Leifker FR, Patterson TL, Heaton RK, Harvey PD. Validating measures of real-world outcome: the results of the VALERO Expert Survey and RAND Appropriateness Panel. *Schizophr Bull.* 2011;37:334-343.

10 Kleinman L, Lieberman J, Dube S, et al. Development and psychometric performance of the schizophrenia objective functioning instrument: an interviewer administered measure of function. *Schizophr Res.* 2009;107:275-285.

11 Morosini PL, Magliano L, Brambilla L, Ugolini S, Pioli R. Development, reliability and acceptability of a new version of the DSM-IV Social and Occupational Functioning Assessment Scale (SOFAS) to assess routine social functioning. *Acta Psychiat Scand.* 2000;101:323-329.

12 Harvey PD, Raykov T, Twamley EM, Vella L, Heaton RK, Patterson TL. Validating the Measurement of Real-World Functional Outcomes: phase I results of the VALERO study. *Am J Psychiatry.* 2011;168:1195-1201.

13 Patterson TL, Goldman S, McKibbin CL, Hughs T, Jeste DV. UCSD Performance-based Skills Assessment: development of a new measure of everyday functioning for severely mentally ill adults. *Schizophr Bull.* 2001;27:235-245.

14 Velligan DI, Diamond P, Glahn DC, et al. The reliability and validity of the Test of Adaptive Behavior in Schizophrenia (TABS). *Psychiatry Res.* 2007;151:55-66.

15 Loeb PA. *Independent Living Scales Manual.* San Antonio, TX: The Psychological Corporation; 1996.

16 Green MF, Schooler NR, Kern RD, et al. Evaluation of functionally meaningful measures for clinical trials of cognition enhancement in schizophrenia. *Am J Psychiatry.* 2001;168:400-407.

5. Quality of life measurements in a person with schizophrenia

George Awad

'Quality of life' over the past few decades has emerged as a significant construct, reflecting a new image of health as viewed from a biopsychosocial perspective. Quality of life assessments have been increasingly used as an important attribute in patient care, in cost–utility analysis of clinical interventions and program comparisons, in resource allocations and for policy decision making.

Historically, interest in quality of life in schizophrenia coincided with the mounting concerns about the state of the chronically mentally ill in the community following the precipitous deinstitutionalization of patients in the early 1960s to a community that lacked resources and was not ready to receive them. As the construct of quality of life in schizophrenia gained currency and popularity, extensive research interest focused on the measurement of quality of life and the development of assessment tools for such measurement [1].

Scales for measurement of quality of life in schizophrenia

The literature relating to quality of life scaling in schizophrenia is crowded with a large number of proposed scales. The scales included in this brief and selective review, are those in common use, those that have proven or promising utility as well as of known psychometrics. Extensive reviews of all available scales have been published previously [1,2].

Disease-specific quality of life scales

Satisfaction with Life Domains Scale

The Satisfaction with Life Domains Scale (SLDS) [3] is a 15-item self-report scale that covers physical, social, economic, and psychological functioning domains. It takes approximately 15 minutes to complete and has good psychometrics. However, the test–retest reliability is not known.

Quality of Life Interview

The Quality of Life Interview (QoLI) [4] is structured into 143 items administered by a trained interviewer. It covers physical, economic, social, and psychological functioning, as well as medical and psychiatric care during the previous year. The scale takes approximately 45–60 minutes to

R. Keefe (ed.), *Guide to Assessment Scales in Schizophrenia*,
DOI: 10.1007/978-1-908517-71-5_5,
© Springer Healthcare, a part of Springer Science+Business Media 2012

administer and has good psychometrics. A recent, brief version includes 74 items as well as the addition of a subjective component. The QoLI is a good scale for long-term studies and is well suited for rehabilitation studies. However, it remains to be demonstrated if this scale has the sensitivity to detect the small changes necessary for short or intermediate drug studies.

Quality of Life Scale

The Quality of Life Scale (QLS) [5] is a semi-structured interview, comprising 21 items. It requires a trained clinician and takes approximately 45 minutes to administer. The QLS covers four domains:
1. Intrapsychic foundations.
2. Interpersonal relations.
3. Instrumental role.
4. Common objects and activities.

It has good internal consistency, test–retest and inter-observer reliability, but there are inconsistent data about convergent validity.

The QLS was initially introduced as a checklist for the assessment of deficit symptoms in schizophrenia and as such the scale is more reflective of the presence of negative and deficit symptoms rather than a specific assessment tool for quality of life. However, two of its domains (the instrumental role and common objects and activities) are relevant to quality of life assessments.

Lancashire Quality of Life Profile

The Lancashire Quality of Life Profile (LQoLP) [6] is a structured interview that includes 105 items that cover nine domains:
1. Work/education.
2. Leisure/participation.
3. Religion.
4. Finances.
5. Living situation.
6. Legal/safety.
7. Family relations.
8. Social relations.
9. Health.

The interviewer does require some training and the scale administration takes approximately 50 minutes. This scale has good psychometrics.

Subjective Quality of Life Analysis

The Subjective Quality of Life Analysis (S.QUA.L.A.) [7] is a recently introduced multidimensional questionnaire. It is self-administered and covers 22 domains ranging from traditional life concern such as food, family, and relations but also assesses more abstract issues such as political, justice, freedom, truth, beauty, art, and love. Every item is assessed based on the degree of satisfaction, and the S.QUA.L.A. has good psychometrics.

Quality of Life Questionnaire

The Quality of Life Questionnaire (S-QUOL-41) [8] is self-administered, multidimensional, and consists of 41 items arranged in eight subscales:

1. Psychological wellbeing.
2. Self-esteem.
3. Family relationships.
4. Relationships with friends.
5. Resilience.
6. Physical wellbeing.
7. Autonomy.
8. Sentimental life.

The administration time of the S-QUOL-41 is not known. It has good psychometrics and high internal consistency, reproducibility, and responsiveness. A short version, S-QUOL-18, that comprises 18 items has been recently introduced.

Schizophrenia Quality of Life Scale

The Schizophrenia Quality of Life Scale (SQLS) [9] consists of 30 items. It is a self-report-style assessment, and is organized into three subscales:

- psychosocial;
- motivation and energy; and
- symptoms and side effects.

The SQLS takes 10 minutes to complete and has good psychometrics. Although it is not widely used at present, it was recently validated for Chinese-speaking populations in Singapore [10].

Generic quality of life scales

SF-36 Health Survey

The SF-36 Health Survey [11] includes eight subscales:

1. Physical functioning.
2. Physical role.
3. Bodily pain.
4. General health.
5. Emotional problems.
6. Social functioning.
7. Vitality.
8. Mental health.

The SF-36 can be self- or interviewer-administered, is suitable for computerized administration, and has good psychometrics. Physical health items are well represented in this scale.

Global Scale of Adaptive Functioning

The range of the Global Scale of Adaptive Functioning (GAF) [12] is between 1 and 100, with 1 representing the most ill individual, hypothetically, and 100 representing the healthiest. The scale is divided into ten equal segments.

The GAF has good psychometrics, has been extensively tested, has good reliability and sensitivity to change, good concurrent and predictive validity, and good inter-rater reliability. The major limitation of GAF is that the ratings are based not only on overall functioning but also incorporates severity of symptoms.

Purpose-specific quality of life scales

Drug Attitude Inventory

The Drug Attitude Inventory [13] is a 30-item self-report inventory (DAI-30), that assesses the subjective impacts of antipsychotic medication. A shorter, ten-item questionnaire exists (DAI-10), which takes less than 10 minutes to complete. The DAI-30 has good psychometrics and the DAI-10 retains the basic psychometrics of the DAI-30.

The scale has been extensively used in clinical trials of antipsychotic medications, and has become the 'gold standard' for development of other scales in the area. The DAI-30 has good predictive validity for medication adherence behavior.

Personal Evaluation of Transition in Treatment

The Personal Evaluation of Transition in Treatment (PETiT) [14] is a 30-item self-administered assessment and takes approximately 5–10 minutes to complete. Designed to capture aspects of subjective responses to, and tolerability of, antipsychotic medications, treatment adherence, and the impact of antipsychotic drug therapy on quality of life, the PETiT has good psychometrics and is frequently used in clinical trials of antipsychotic medications as well as in studies of transition in treatment from one medication to another.

Impact of Weight on Quality of Life – Lite

The Impact of Weight on Quality of Life – Lite (IWQOL-Lite) [15] is a 30-item self-report tool assessing the quality of life related to body weight. It is arranged in five subscales:
1. Physical function.
2. Self esteem.
3. Sexual life.
4. Work.
5. Public distress.

The IWQOL-Lite has good psychometrics and a good correlation with body mass index (BMI).

Body Weight Image and Self-Esteem Evaluation Questionnaire

The Body Weight Image and Self-Esteem Evaluation Questionnaire (B-WISE) [16] is a 12-item self-reported scale, that assesses the psychological and psychosocial impact of weight gain associated with psychotropic drug use. It has good psychometrics, is sensitive to change in body weight and correlates with BMI.

Important considerations when using scales

Important issues to recognize and be aware of when using these scales and assessments are [17]:

- Though the basic construct of quality of life is subjective in nature, it also includes an objective component.
- Quality of life in schizophrenia is multidimensional and needs to be reflected in its assessment.
- Quality of life needs to be assessed in the context of total human experience noting the impact of the affective and cognitive state on self-assessment.
- Quality of life is not expected to change quickly; an appropriate time-framework needs to be recognized.
- Measurement of quality of life by itself is not enough until the next step is taken, which is integrating quality of life data in care plans.

References

1   Awad AG, Voruganti LNP. Measuring quality of life in patients with schizophrenia. *Pharmacoeconomics*. 1997;11:32-47.
2   Awad AG, Voruganti LNP. Measuring quality of life in schizophrenia: an update. *Pharmacoeconomics*. 2012;30:183-195.
3   Baker F, Intagliata J. Quality of life in the evaluation of community support systems. *Eval Program Plann*. 1982;5:69-79.
4   Lehman AF. A quality of life interview for the chronically mentally ill. *Eval Program Plann*. 1988;11:51-62.
5   Heinrichs DW, Hanlon TE, Carpenter WT. The Quality of Life Scale: an instrument for rating the schizophrenic deficit symptoms. *Schizophr Bull*. 1984;10:388-398.
6   Oliver JPJ. How to use quality of life measures in individual care. In: Priebe S, Oliver JPJ, Kaiser W, eds. *Quality of Life and Mental Health Care*. Petersfield, UK: Wrightson Biomedical Publishing; 1999:81-105.
7   Nadalet L, Kohl FS, Pringuey D, et al. Validation of a Subjective Quality of Life Questionnaire (S.QUA.LA) in schizophrenia. *Schizophr Res*. 2005;76:73-81.
8   Auquier P, Simioni MC, Sapin C, et al. Development and validation of a patient-based health related quality of life questionnaire in schizophrenia: the S-QOL. *Schizophr Res*. 2003;63:137-149.
9   Wilkinson G, Hesdon B, Wild D, et al. Self-report quality of life measure for people with schizophrenia: SQLS. *Br J Psychiatry*. 2000;177:42-46.
10 Luo N, Seng BK, Xie F, Li SC, Thumboo J. Psychometric evaluation of the Schizophrenia Quality of Life Scale (SQLS) in English- and Chinese-speaking Asians in Singapore. *Qual Life Res*. 2008;17:115-122.
11 Ware JE, Sherbourne CD. The MOS 36-Item Short Form Health Status Survey (SF-36). 1. Conceptual framework and item selection. *Med Care*. 1992;30:MS253-MS265.

12 Endicott J, Spitzer RL, Fleiss Jl. The Global Assessment Scale: a procedure for measuring overall severity of psychiatric disturbance. *Arch Gen Psychiatry* 1976;33:766-771.

13 Awad AG. Subjective response to neuroleptics in schizophrenia. *Schizophr Bull.* 1993;19:609-618.

14 Voruganti LNP, Awad AG. Personal evaluation of transition in treatment (PETiT): a scale to measure subjective aspects of antipsychotic drug therapy in schizophrenia. *Schizophr Res.* 2002;56:37-46.

15 Kolotkin RL, Crosby RD, Corey-Lisle PK, et al. Performance of weight-related measure of quality of life in a psychiatric sample. *Qual Life Res.* 2006;15:587-596.

16 Awad AG, Voruganti LNP. Body weight, image and self-esteem evaluation questionnaire: development and validation of a new scale. *Schizophr Res.* 2004;70:63-67.

17 Awad AG, Voruganti LNP. Antipsychotic medications, schizophrenia and the issue of quality of life. In: Ritsner M, Awad AG (eds). *Quality of Life Impairment in Schizophrenia, Mood and Anxiety Disorders.* The Netherlands: Springer; 2007:307-319.

6. Antipsychotic side-effect rating scales in schizophrenia

Mark Taylor

Antipsychotic adverse side effects

Adverse 'side' effects are documented in all licensed antipsychotic medications, although the precise nature and severity of these side effects is variable. The most commonly encountered antipsychotic-related side effects seen in everyday clinical practice are those of sedation, weight gain, tremor or neuromuscular stiffness, and a dry mouth. A summary of the major evidence-based adverse side effects of the most commonly used antipsychotic medications is depicted in Table 6.1 [1].

Clinicians have generally thought that first-generation antipsychotics (FGA) are associated with extrapyramidal side effects (EPS) (Table 6.1), whereas second-generation antipsychotics (SGA) are commonly associated with metabolic problems, particularly weight gain and prolactin elevation [2,3]. However, in the aftermath of the CATIE trials [4] it has become increasingly clear that the 'typical' or FGA versus 'atypical' or SGA dichotomy was not necessarily valid in terms of both efficacy and side-effect profiles. For example, newer agents like aripiprazole or high-dose risperidone can lead to akathisia (EPS) [5,6], whereas haloperidol can elevate prolactin and lead to sexual dysfunction [7] and chlorpromazine can cause weight gain [8].

Side-effect or adverse-effect rating scales for schizophrenia

A nonsystematic search for all published rating scales for the adverse side effects of medication used in schizophrenia was carried out, including PubMed® and Google Scholar® searches, citation checking, and consulting national experts. This search was conducted in August 2011 and identified 24 separate side-effect rating scales published since 1970, with five being developed as self-rating scales. Of these 24 scales, 16 had published data on reliability and/or validity, although the search was unable find the validation data on the Abnormal Involuntary Movement Scale (AIMS) [9] and the Yale Extrapyramidal Symptoms Scale (YESS) [10], even though this is referred to elsewhere. These 16 validated scales are summarized and reviewed in Tables 6.2 [9,11–19] and 6.3 [10,20–26]. Scales that have been validated for EPS and drug-induced parkinsonism and metabolic side effects are presented in Table 6.4 [9–24].

R. Keefe (ed.), *Guide to Assessment Scales in Schizophrenia*,
DOI: 10.1007/978-1-908517-71-5_6,
© Springer Healthcare, a part of Springer Science+Business Media 2012

Table 6.1 A guide to the relative side effects of antipsychotics

	EPS	Prolactin elevation	Weight gain	QTc prolongation	Sedation	Hypotension	Anticholinergic effects
Amisulpride	+	+++	+	+	-/+	-	-
Aripiprazole	+/-	-	+/-	-	-/+	-	-
Chlorpromazine	++	+++	++/+++	++	+++	+++	++/+++
Clozapine	-	-	+++	+	+++	+++	+++
Haloperidol	+++	+++	+	+++	+	+	+
Olanzapine	+/-	+	+++	+	++	+	+
Paliperidone	+	+++	+/++	+	+	+/++	+/-
Perphenazine	+++	+++	++	-/+	+/++	+	+
Quetiapine	-	-	++	+	++	++	+
Risperidone	+/++	+++	++	+	+	+/++	+/-
Sulpiride	+	++	+	+	+	-	+
Trifluoperazine	+++	+++	+/++	++	+	+	+/-
Zotepine	+	+++	++/+++	+/++	++/+++	++	+

The extrapyramidal side effects (EPS) include akathisia, dystonias, parkinsonism, and tardive dyskinesia. QTc, QT interval corrected for heart rate; +++, frequent side effects at therapeutic dose; ++, sometimes causes side effects at therapeutic dose; +, mild or occasional side effects at therapeutic dose; –, little risk or minimal side effects at therapeutic dose. Data from NICE [1]. © National Institute for Health and Clinical Excellence, reproduced with permission.

Interestingly, some of the better-known scales revealed by our search do not specifically assess medication-induced side effects, such as the Drug Attitude Inventory (DAI-10) [13], the Subjective Well-being under Neuroleptic (SWN) treatment scale [27], and the Subjects' Reaction to Antipsychotics (SRA) questionnaire [28].

The Glasgow Antipsychotic Side-effect Scale

The Glasgow Antipsychotic Side-effect Scale (GASS) is a relatively recent addition to the choice of scales assessing antipsychotic-induced side effects (Figure 6.1) [15]. The GASS includes ratings of both neuromuscular and metabolic side effects (after literature review and physician and patient focus-group feedback) and can be a patient self-completion tool. The GASS rates both frequency and severity of any side effects. The scale was calibrated against the Liverpool University Neuroleptic Side-Effect Rating Scale (LUNSERS) [17] in 50 outpatients on SGA, compared to 50 healthy individuals not on antipsychotics, and was found to have good discriminatory power; construct validity; and test–retest reliability. The GASS is quick to complete, either for the clinician or patient, and the use of plain English helps comprehension. It is independent of any commercial interest and can be used without cost. A spreadsheet graph maker for the GASS, useful to illustrate trends over time, is available freely from the author on request.

Table 6.2 Comparison and critique of the most commonly used side-effect scales

Scale	Completed by?	Focus	Number of questions	Approx. time taken (mins)
Abnormal Involuntary Movement Scale (AIMS)	Clinician	EPS	12	10
Antipsychotic Non-Neurological Side Effect Rating Scale (ANNSERS)	Clinician and self-rated	Global	35	30
Barnes Akathisia Rating Scale (BARS)	Clinician and self-rated	Akathisia	4	10
Drug Attitude Inventory (DAI)	Self	Attitudes	30	10
Extrapyramidal Symptom Rating Scale (ESRS)	Clinician	EPS	13	15
Glasgow Antipsychotic Side-effect Scale (GASS)	Self	Global	22	10
Hillside Akathisia Scale (HAS)	Clinician and self-rated	Akathisia	5	10
Liverpool University Neuroleptic Side-Effect Rating Scale (LUNSERS)	Self	Global	51	20
Simpson-Angus Scale (SAS)	Clinician	EPS	10	10
Udvalg for Kliniske Undersøgelser Side-Effect Rating Scale (UKUSERS)	Clinician	EPS	48	30

(continues overleaf).

Table 6.2 Comparison and critique of the most commonly used side-effect scales (continued)

Scale	Reference	Advantages	Disadvantages
Abnormal Involuntary Movement Scale (AIMS)	Guy (1976) [9]	Quick and easy to use Objective rating of EPS	Only assesses EPS
Antipsychotic Non-Neurological Side Effect Rating Scale (ANNSERS)	Yusufi et al (2005) [11]	Wide range of FGA and SGA side effects covered	Lengthy and time consuming
Barnes Akathisia Rating Scale (BARS)	Barnes (1989) [12]	Quick Used extensively in trials Subjective and objective components	Only assesses akathisia
Drug Attitude Inventory (DAI)	Hogan et al (1983) [13]	Easy to use and understand Examines attitude/ adherence	Not specifically for side effects
Extrapyramidal Symptom Rating Scale (ESRS)	Chouinard et al (1980) [14]	Objective rating of EPS	Only assesses EPS Does not differentiate between dyskinesia and dystonia
Glasgow Antipsychotic Side-effect Scale (GASS)	Waddell & Taylor (2008) [15]	Quick and easy to use and understand Covers a wide range of FGA and SGA side effects	Validated only in those on SGA
Hillside Akathisia Scale (HAS)	Fleischhaker et al (1989) [16]	Easy to use Subjective and objective components	Only assesses akathisia
Liverpool University Neuroleptic Side-Effect Rating Scale (LUNSERS)	Day et al (1995) [17]	Easy to use Subjective and objective components	Time consuming One word symptoms can be difficult for patients to understand
Simpson-Angus Scale (SAS)	Simpson & Angus (1970) [18]	Quick objective rating of EPS Used extensively in trials	Only assesses EPS Some items (eg, head drop) difficult to score
Udvalg for Kliniske Undersøgelser Side-Effect Rating Scale (UKUSERS)	Lingjaerde et al (1987) [19]	Comprehensive	Lengthy interview and observation Only assesses neurological effects Reliability and validity data limited

(continued). EPS, Extrapyramidal side effects; FGA, first-generation antipsychotics; SGA, second-generation antipsychotics. Data from [9,11–19].

Table 6.3 Comparison and critique of less frequently used side-effect scales

Scale	Reference	Number of questions	Approx. time taken (mins)	Completed by?	Focus	Advantages	Disadvantages
Drug-Induced Extrapyramidal Symptoms Scale (DIEPSS)	Inada (1996) [20]	9	10	Clinician	EPS	Good inter-rater reliability and agreement with SAS	Only assesses EPS
Maryland Psychiatric Research Center Scale (MPRC)	Cassady et al (1997) [21]	28	30	Clinician	EPS and parkinsonism	Good inter-rater reliability Very detailed	Only assesses involuntary movements
Schedule for Assessment of Drug-Induced Movement Disorders (SADIMoD)	Loonen et al (2001) [22]	Numerous	60	Clinician	EPS	Combines other scales including AIMS [3], BARS [6], MADRS [19], and PANSS [20] Highly detailed	Complex and time consuming
St Hans Rating Scale (SHRS)	Gerlach et al (1993) [23]	4 blocks, each 7 points	15	Trained clinician	EPS	Good validity and reliability	Only assesses EPS Unclear interpretation of scores
Yale Extrapyramidal Side-effects Scale (YESS)	Mazure et al (1995) [10]	8	10	Clinician	EPS	Brief, easy to use Good reliability	Only assesses EPS Validated against Parkinson's disease
United Parkinson Disease Rating Scale (UPDRS)	Goetz et al (2003) [24]	44	30	Clinician	Parkinsonism	Widely used in Parkinson's disease Some mental state/function questions	Not designed for drug-induced states Lengthy

AIMS, Abnormal Involuntary Movement Scale; BARS, Barnes Akathisia Rating Scale; EPS, extrapyramidal side effects; MADRS, Montgomery-Åsberg Depression Rating Scale; PANSS, Positive and Negative Syndrome Scale; SAS, Simpson Angus Scale. Data from [10,20–24].

Table 6.4 **Scales validated for EPS, drug-induced parkinsonism, and metabolic side-effects**

Scale	Reference	Validated for EPS and drug-induced parkinsonism?	Validated for metabolic side effects?
Abnormal Involuntary Movement Scale (AIMS)	Guy (1976) [9]	Yes	No
Antipsychotic Non-Neurological Side Effect Rating Scale (ANNSERS)	Yusufi et al (2005) [11]	Yes	Yes
Barnes Akathisia Rating Scale (BARS)	Barnes (1989) [12]	Yes	No
Drug-Induced Extrapyramidal Symptoms Scale (DIEPSS)	Inada (1996) [20]	Yes	No
Extrapyramidal Symptom Rating Scale (ESRS)	Chouinard et al (1980) [14]	Yes	No
Glasgow Antipsychotic Side-effect Scale* (GASS)	Waddell & Taylor (2008) [15]	Yes	Yes
Hillside Akathisia Scale (HAS)	Fleischhaker et al (1989) [16]	Yes	No
Liverpool University Neuroleptic Side-Effect Rating Scale* (LUNSERS)	Day et al (1995) [17]	Yes	Yes
Maryland Psychiatric Research Center Scale (MPRC)	Cassady et al (1997) [21]	Yes	No
Schedule for Assessment of Drug-Induced Movement Disorders (SADIMoD)	Loonen et al (2001) [24]	Yes	No
Simpson-Angus Scale (SAS)	Simpson & Angus (1970) [18]	Yes	No
St Hans Rating Scale* (SHRS)	Gerlach et al (1993) [23]	Yes	No
Udvalg for Kliniske Undersøgelser Side-Effect Rating Scale (UKUSERS)	Lingjaerde et al (1987) [19]	Yes	No
United Parkinson Disease Rating Scale (UPDRS)	Goetz et al (2003) [24]	Yes	No
Yale Extrapyramidal Side-effects Scale (YESS)	Mazure et al (1995) [10]	Yes	No

EPS, extrapyramidal side effects. *Self-rating scale. Data from [9–24].

Figure 6.1 **Glasgow Antipsychotic Side-effect Scale**

Name:

| Age: | Sex: male/female |

Please list current medication and total daily doses below:

This questionnaire is about how you have been recently. It is being used to determine if you are suffering from excessive side effects from your antipsychotic medication.

Please place a tick in the column which best indicates the degree to which you have experienced the following side effects. Tick the end box if you found that the side effect distressed you.

Over the past week	Never	Once	A few times	Every-day	Tick this box if distressing*
1. I felt sleepy during the day					
2. I felt drugged or like a zombie					
3. I felt dizzy when I stood up and/or have fainted					
4. I have felt my heart beating irregularly or unusually fast					
5. My muscles have been tense or jerky					
6. My hands or arms have been shaky					
7. My legs have felt restless and/or I couldn't sit still					
8. I have been drooling					
9. My movements or walking have been slower than usual					
10. I have had, or people have noticed, uncontrollable movements of my face or body					
11. My vision has been blurry					
12. My mouth has been dry					
13. I have had difficulty passing urine					
14. I have felt like I am going to be sick or have vomited					
15. I have wet the bed					
16. I have been very thirsty and/or passing urine frequently					
17. The areas around my nipples have been sore and swollen					
18. I have noticed fluid coming from my nipples					
19. I have had problems enjoying sex					
20. **Men only:** I have had problems getting an erection					

(continues overleaf).

Figure 6.1 **Glasgow Antipsychotic Side-effect Scale** (continued)

Tick **yes or no** for the following questions about the last 3 months	Yes	No	Tick this box if distressing*
21. **Women only:** I have noticed a change in my periods			
22. **Men and women:** I have been gaining weight			
Staff information			
1. Allow the patient to fill in the questionnaire themselves. Questions 1–20 relate to the previous week and Questions 21 and 22 to the last 3 months.			
2. Scoring: For questions 1–20 award 1 point for the answer 'once,' 2 points for the answer 'a few times,' and 3 points for the answer 'everyday.' Please note 0 points are awarded for an answer of 'never.' For Question 21 and 22 award 3 points for a 'yes' answer and 0 points for a 'no.' Total for all questions _____.			
3. For male and female patients a **total score** of: 0–12 Absent/mild side effects. 13–26 Moderate side effects. >26 Severe side effects.			

(continued).*The column relating to the distress experienced with a particular side effect is not scored, but is intended to inform the clinician of the service user's views and condition. Data from Waddell & Taylor [15]. ©2008, reproduced with permission from the British Association for Psychopharmacology.

Acknowledgments

The author thanks Jamie McGowan and Maxine X Patel.

References

1   NHS England National Prescribing Centre. Patient decision aid: antipsychotic drugs. Available at: www.npc.nhs.uk/therapeutics/cns/schizophrenia/resources/pda_schizophrenia.pdf. Accessed April 2, 2012.

2   Peluso MJ, Lewis SW, Barnes TRE, Jones PB. Extrapyramidal motor side-effects of first- and second-generation antipsychotic drugs. *Br J Psychiatry*. [Epub ahead of print March 22, 2012.]

3   Rummel-Kluge C, Komossa K, Schwarz S, et al. Second-generation antipsychotic drugs and extrapyramidal side effects. A systematic review and meta-analysis of head-to-head comparisons. *Schizophr Bull*. 2012;38:167-177.

4   Lieberman JA, Stroup TS, McEvoy JP, et al. Effectiveness of antipsychotic drugs in patients with chronic schizophrenia. *N Engl J Med*. 2005;353:1209-1223.

5   Berman RM, Marcus RN, Swanink R, et al. The efficacy and safety of aripiprazole as adjunctive therapy in major depressive disorder: a multicenter, randomized, double-blind, placebo-controlled study. *J Clin Psychiatry*. 2007;68:843-853.

6   Jayaram MB, Hosalli P, Stroup S. Risperidone versus olanzapine for schizophrenia. *Cochrane Database Syst Rev*. 2006;(2):CD005237.

7   La Torre D, Falorni A. Pharmacological causes of hyperprolactinemia. *Ther Clin Risk Manag*. 2007;3:929-951.

8   Ganguli R. Weight gain associated with antipsychotic drugs. *J Clin Psychiatry*. 1999;60:20-24.

9   Guy WA, ed. Abnormal Involuntary Movement Scale (AIMS). In: *ECDEU Assessment Manual for Psychopharmacology*. Washington, DC: US Department of Health Education and Welfare; 1976:534-537.

10 Mazure CM, Cellar JS, Bowers MB, Nelson JC, Takeshita J, Zigun B. Assessment of extrapyramidal symptoms during acute neuroleptic treatment. *J Clin Psychiatry*. 1995;56:94-100.

11 Yusufi BZ, Mukherjee S, Aitchison K, Dunn G, Page E, Barnes TRE. Inter-rater reliability of the Antipsychotic Non-Neurological Side-Effects Rating Scale (ANNSERS). *Schizophr Bull*. 2005;31:574.

12 Barnes TR. A rating scale for drug-induced akathisia. *Br J Psychiatry*. 1989;154:672-676.

13 Hogan TP, Awad AG, Eastwood R. A self-report scale predictive of drug compliance in schizophrenics: reliability and discriminative validity. *Psychol Med*. 1983;13:177-183.

14 Chouinard G, Ross-Chouinard A, Annable L, Jones B. The Extrapyramidal Symptom Rating Scale. *Can J Neurol Sci*. 1980;7:233.

15 Waddell L, Taylor M. A new self-rating scale for detecting atypical or second generation antipsychotic side effects. *J Psychopharmacol*. 2008:22;238-243.

16 Fleischhacker WW, Bergmann KJ, Perovich R, et al. The Hillside Akathisia Scale: a new rating instrument for neuroleptic induced akathisia. *Psychopharmacol Bull*. 1989;25:222-226.

17 Day JC, Wood G, Dewey M, Bentall RP. A self-rating scale for measuring neuroleptic side-effects. Validation in a group of schizophrenic patients. *Br J Psychiatry*. 1995;166:650-653.

18 Janno S, Holi MM, Tuisku K, Wahlbeck K. Validity of Simpson-Angus Scale (SAS) in a naturalistic schizophrenia population. *BMC Neurol*. 2005;5:5.

19 Lingjaerde O, Ahlfors UG, Bech P, Dencker SJ, Elgen K. The UKU side effect rating scale. A new comprehensive rating scale for psychotropic drugs and a cross-sectional study of side effects in neuroleptic-treated patients. *Acta Psychiatr Scand Suppl*. 1987;334:1-100.

20 Inada T, Yagi G. Current topics in tardive dyskinesia in Japan. *Psychiatry Clin Neurosci*. 1995;49:239-244.

21 Cassady SL, Thaker GK, Summerfelt A, Tamminga CA. The Maryland Psychiatric Research Center Scale and the characterization of involuntary movements. *Psychiatry Res*. 1997;18:21-37.

22 Loonen AJM, Doorschot CH, van Hemert DA, Oostelbos MCM, Sijben AES. The Schedule for the Assessment of Drug-Induced Movement Disorders (SADIMoD): inter-rater reliability and construct validity. *Int J Neuropsychopharmacol*. 2001;4:347-360.

23 Gerlach J, Korgard S. The St. Hans Rating Scale for the extrapyramidal symptoms: reliability and validity. *Acta Psychiatr Scand*. 1993;87:244-252.

24 Goetz CG, Poewe W, Rascol O, et al; the Movement Disorder Society Task Force. The Unified Parkinson's Disease Rating Scale (UPDRS): status and recommendations. *Mov Disord*. 2003;18:738-750.

25 Montgomery SA, Asberg M. A new depression scale designed to be sensitive to change. *Br J Psychiatry*. 1979;134:382-389.

26 Kay S, Fiszbein A, Opler L. The Positive and Negative Syndrome Scale (PANSS) for Schizophrenia. *Schizophr Bull*. 1987;13:261-276.

27 Naber, D. A self-rating to measure subjective effects of neuroleptic drugs, relationships to objective psychopathology, quality of life, compliance and other clinical variables. *Int Clin Psychopharmacol*. 1995;10:133-138.

28 Wolters HA, Knegtering R, Wiersma D, van den Bosch RJ. Evaluation of the subjects' response to antipsychotics questionnaire. *Int Clin Psychopharmacol*. 2006;21:63-69.

7. Assessment scales for insight

Insight forms part of the routine evaluation of all psychiatric patients but is particularly relevant to those with schizophrenia. Over the last 20 years there has been an explosion of interest in the concept of 'insight' and this has coincided with the development of a number of scales and assessment instruments. The term is often used interchangeable with 'awareness of illness' and lack of insight is frequently termed 'denial.' The construct has predictive validity in terms of a variety of functional outcomes [1] and treatment adherence [2]. Insight is related rather modestly to psychopathology [3]; poor insight tends to be associated with cognitive impairment [4,5] and, in some more recent studies, reductions in regional brain volumes [6,7].

The challenge of coming up with a satisfactory definition of insight motivated the development of assessment scales, which in turn shaped our understanding of the construct. Hence an insight score automatically implies that it is a dimension rather than 'all or none.' Furthermore, the most widely used scales are explicitly multidimensional – formalizing the view that insight has different aspects that may vary somewhat independently.

Measuring insight

Positive and Negative Syndrome Scale
The Positive and Negative Syndrome Scale (PANSS) contains a general item (G12), which measures 'lack of judgment and insight' [8] on a scale of 1–7, where a higher score represents lower insight (Figure 7.1).

Insight and Treatment Attitudes Questionnaire
The Insight and Treatment Attitudes Questionnaire (ITAQ) [9,10] is an 11-item clinician-rated scale (scored 0, 1, 2) based on a two-dimensional definition of insight (Figure 7.2). The scale measures the extent to which a patient judges their aberrant experiences to be pathological in a manner similar to mental health professionals, and the extent to which patients feel they need treatment, which may include medication or hospitalization.

R. Keefe (ed.), _Guide to Assessment Scales in Schizophrenia_,
DOI: 10.1007/978-1-908517-71-5_7,
© Springer Healthcare, a part of Springer Science+Business Media 2012

55

Figure 7.1 **Positive and Negative Syndrome Scale**

1. Absent	Definition does not apply.
2. Minimal	Questionable pathology; may be at the upper extreme of normal limits.
3. Mild	Recognizes having a psychiatric disorder but clearly underestimates its seriousness, the implication for treatment, or the importance of taking measures to avoid relapse. Future planning may be poorly conceived.
4. Moderate	Patient shows only a vague or shallow recognition of illness. There may be fluctuations in acknowledgement of being ill or little awareness of major symptoms that are present, such as delusions, disorganized thinking, suspiciousness, and social withdrawal. The patient may rationalize the need for treatment in terms of its relieving lesser symptoms, such as anxiety, tension, and sleep difficulty.
5. Moderate–severe	Acknowledges past but not present psychiatric disorder. If challenged, the patient may concede the presence of some unrelated or insignificant symptoms, which tend to be explained away by gross misinterpretation or delusional thinking. The need for psychiatric treatment similarly goes unrecognized.
6. Severe	Patient denies ever having had a psychiatric disorder. They disavow the presence of any psychiatric symptoms in the past or present and, though compliant, denies the need for treatment and hospitalization.
7. Extreme	Emphatic denial of past and present psychiatric illness. Current hospitalization and treatment are given a delusional interpretation (eg, punishment for misdeeds, as persecution by tormentors, etc) and the patient may thus refuse to cooperate with therapists, medication, or other aspects of treatment.

The PANSS G12 item measures 'lack of judgment and insight.' Data from Kay et al [8]. ©1987, Oxford University Press.

Figure 7.2 **Insight and Treatment Attitudes Questionnaire**

Questions asked of chronic schizophrenic patients to determine their degree of insight into their illness:

1. At the time of your admission, did you need to come to the hospital?
2. At the time of your admission, were you ill in any way or was there any way in which you were not normal?
3. At the time of your admission, was anything the matter with your mind?
4. Are you receiving medication (pills)?
5. Do you still need treatment now?
6. Are you ill in any way now, or is there any way in which you are not normal?
7. Is there anything the matter with your mind now; do you have a mental illness?
8. Do you believe you need to take 'nerve medicine' or medicine for a mental illness?
9. Does the medicine you take here do you any good?
10. Does the medicine you take here do you any harm?
11. When you are discharged, will you need to take medication?

Answers are scored as follows: 2, good response; 1, partial response; 0, no insight. Data from McEvoy et al [9,10]. Reproduced with permission from Dr J McEvoy.

Commentary on the Insight and Treatment Attitudes Questionnaire

The scale correlates with symptomatology to a moderate degree, suggesting its distinctiveness but also providing some construct validity. Lower scores are found in involuntary patients. This definition has a greater focus on attitudes toward treatment rather than psychopathology, which must be taken into account before using it for research.

Schedule for the Assessment of Insight – Expanded version

The Schedule for the Assessment of Insight – Expanded version (SAI-E) [11] is a 12-item semi-structured interview (Figure 7.3), including three items addressing compliance to treatment (Figure 7.1). The SAI-E builds upon its predecessor, the Schedule for the Assessment of Insight [12,13], a seven-item assessment based on the same three factors:

- recognition of having a mental illness (items 1–5);
- ability to relabel symptoms as abnormal (items 7 and 8); and
- compliance with treatment (items 6, A and B).

As well as this, there is an item assessing 'hypothetical contradiction' (item 9), which refers to a patient's reaction if someone were to deny their psychotic experiences, and is usually included with the relabeling items. It also includes a 7-point overall compliance item (the latter not included in the total insight score). These factors can be analyzed independently, or summed to make a total score (0–28).

Completion of the scale does not require special training, although it does assume knowledge of the patient's psychopathology and some experience in eliciting psychotic symptoms, so is best completed by a health care professional alongside a clinical interview or a general psychopathology assessment using an instrument such as the PANSS or Brief Psychiatric Rating Scale (BPRS). The compliance items can be completed from the interview but it is strongly recommended that the rater makes use of information from a professional or informal carer. There is a good level of agreement between the SAI-E and other single- or multi-item measures; Sanz et al [14] found correlation coefficients ranging between 0.85 and 0.91 for several widely used insight scales. High correlations have also been found between the Schedule for the assessment of Unawareness of Mental Disorder (SUMD) and the SAI-E [6]. A principal components factor analysis (with varimax rotation) of the insight data on 116 psychosis patients yielded three factors that accounted for 66.5% of the variance (lowest eigenvalue 1.05) [7]. This finding corresponds directly with the three-component model of insight described above. Ratings of total insight consist of the combined SAI-E scores (items 1–11).

The SAI-E is best used to measure change and to explore correlations with clinical, biological, or psychosocial variables [15], either as a single continuous measure or as separate dimensional measures. It does not have a 'cut-off,' although scores are strongly related to notions of capacity (to make treatment decisions) and a score of less than 15 indicates likely incapacity [16].

Inter-rater reliability of the Schedule for the Assessment of Insight – Expanded version

In one study [7], SAI-E interviewers scored a battery of 16 completed interviews prepared specifically to assess inter-rater reliability. These schedules were verbatim reproductions of real interviews with the scoring sections left blank. Intra-class correlation coefficients for the total SAI-E scores between the raters ranged from 0.92 to 0.98 ($P<0.001$).

Commentary on the Schedule for the Assessment of Insight – Expanded version

The SAI-E is designed to assess insight into psychotic symptoms in relation to the current mental state (eg, hallucinations, delusions and thought disorder). This means that using it to assess retrospective insight, while possible, requires modification, for example "When you were in

Figure 7.3 Schedule for the Assessment of Insight – Expanded version

1. "Do you think you have been experiencing any emotional or psychological changes or difficulties?"	
Often (thought present most of the day, most days) = 2	Score:
Sometimes (thought present occasionally) = 1	
Never (ask why doctors/others think so) = 0	
If brief write verbatim reply, otherwise summarize response. Please add explanatory comments if appropriate:	

2. "Do you think this means there is something wrong with you?" (eg, a nervous condition). If previous answer was "never" or "no" ask: "If the doctor(s) and/or others think you have been experiencing emotional or psychological changes or difficulties do you think there must be something wrong with you even though you don't feel it yourself?"	
Often (thought present most of the day, most days) = 2	Score:
Sometimes (thought present occasionally) = 1	
Never (ask why doctors/others think so) = 0	
If brief write verbatim reply, otherwise summarize response. Please add explanatory comments if appropriate:	

3. "Do you think your condition amounts to a mental illness or mental disorder?"	
Often (thought present most of the day, most days) = 2	Score:
Sometimes (thought present occasionally) = 1	
Never (ask why doctors/others think so) = 0	
If brief write verbatim reply, otherwise summarize response. Please add explanatory comments if appropriate:	

If positive score on previous two items, proceed to 4, otherwise go to item 6

4. "How do you explain your condition/disorder/illness?"	
Reasonable account given based on plausible mechanisms (appropriate given social, cultural, and educational background, eg, excess stress, chemical imbalance, family history, etc) = 2	Score:
Confused account, or overheard explanation without adequate understanding or "don't know" = 1	
Delusional or bizarre explanation = 0	
If brief write verbatim reply, otherwise summarize response. Please add explanatory comments if appropriate:	

If positive score on items 1, 2, and 3, proceed to 5, otherwise go to item 6

(continues opposite).

Figure 7.3 Schedule for the Assessment of Insight – Expanded version (continued)

---

5. "Has your nervous/emotional/psychological/mental/psychiatric condition [use patient's term] led to adverse consequences or problems in your life?" (eg, conflict with others, neglect, financial or accommodation difficulties, irrational, impulsive, or dangerous behavior)

Yes (with example) = 2   Score:

Unsure (cannot give example or contradicts self) = 1

No = 0

If brief write verbatim reply, otherwise summarize response. Please add explanatory comments if appropriate:

---

6. "Do you think your ... condition [use patient's term] or the problem resulting from it warrants (needs) treatment?"

Yes (with plausible reason) = 2   Score:

Unsure (cannot give example or contradicts self) = 1

No = 0

If brief write verbatim reply, otherwise summarize response. Please add explanatory comments if appropriate:

---

7. Pick the most prominent symptoms <u>up to</u> a maximum of four. Then rate awareness of each symptom out of 4 as below. (Interviewer to assess which symptoms to rate from previous interviews eg, highest scoring on the Brief Psychiatric Rating Scale and/or from patient's current presentation)

Examples:
- "Do you think that the belief ... is not real/not really happening (could you be imagining things)?"
- "Do you think the 'voices' you hear are actually real people talking, or is it something arising from your own mind?"
- "Have you been able to think clearly, or do your thoughts seem mixed up/confused? Is your speech jumbled?"
- "Would you say you have been more agitated/overactive/speeded up/withdrawn than usual?"
- "Are you aware of any problem with attention/concentration/memory?"
- "Have you a problem with doing what you intend/getting going/finishing tasks/motivation?"

Symptom 1 – type:		Symptom 2 – type:		Symptom 3 – type:		Symptom 4 – type:	
Rating:		Rating:		Rating:		Rating:	

Definitely (full awareness) = 4   Mean:

Probably (moderate awareness) = 3

Unsure (sometimes yes, sometimes no) = 2

Possibly (slight awareness) = 1

Absolutely not (no awareness) = 0

If brief write verbatim reply, otherwise summarize response. Please add explanatory comments if appropriate:

(continues overleaf).

Figure 7.3 Schedule for the Assessment of Insight – Expanded version (continued)

8. For each symptom rated above (up to a maximum of four), ask patient ... "How do you explain ... (false beliefs, hearing voices, thoughts muddled, lack of drive etc)?"

Symptom 1		Symptom 2		Symptom 3		Symptom 4	
Rating:		Rating:		Rating:		Rating:	

Part of my illness = 4	Mean:
Due to nervous condition = 3	
Reaction to stress/fatigue = 2	
Unsure, maybe one of the above = 1	
Can't say, or delusional/bizarre explanation = 0	

If brief write verbatim reply, otherwise summarize response. Please add explanatory comments if appropriate:

9. "How do you feel when people do not believe you (when you talk about ... delusions or hallucinations)?"

That's when I know I'm sick = 4	Mean:
I wonder whether something's wrong with me = 3	
I'm confused and I don't know what to think = 2	
I'm still sure despite what others say = 1	
They're lying = 0	

If brief write verbatim reply, otherwise summarize response. Please add explanatory comments if appropriate:

After interview go to the end of this form and fill in grid as appropriate.

Compliance to treatment/therapy/medication – patient's primary nurse to rate following three items (A–C)

A. How does patient accept treatment (includes passive acceptance)?

Often (may rarely question need for treatment) = 2	Mean:
Sometimes (may occasionally question need for treatment) = 1	
Never (ask why) = 0	

Please add explanatory comments if appropriate:

B. Does patient ask for treatment unprompted?

Often (excludes inappropriate request for medication, etc) = 2	Mean:
Sometimes (rate here if forgetfulness/disorganization leads to occasional requests only) = 1	
Never (ask why doctors/others think so) = 0	

Please add explanatory comments if appropriate:

(continues opposite).

Figure 7.3 Schedule for the Assessment of Insight – Expanded version (continued)

C. Summary of compliance to treatment/therapy/medication

Complete refusal = 1	Mean:
Partial refusal (eg, refusing depot drugs or accepting only the minimum dose) = 2	
Reluctant acceptance (accepting only because treatment is compulsory or questioning the need for treatment often, eg, every 2 days) = 3	
Occasional reluctance about treatment (questioning the need for treatment once a week) = 4	
Passive acceptance = 5	
Moderate participation (some knowledge of and interest in treatment and no prompting needed to take the drugs) = 6	
Active participation (ready acceptance, and taking some responsibility for treatment) = 7	

Please add explanatory comments if appropriate:

Please complete this grid (as appropriate)

	Patient	Primary Nurse
ID		
Date of interview		
Time started		
Time finished		
Rater ID		
Score summary		
1:		
2:		
3:		
4:		
5:		
6:		
7: (mean)		
8: (mean)		
9:		
Sub total:		
A:		
B:		
Total:	Item C:	

*NB: Item C **is not** combined with other scores*

General comments/observations:

(continued). Data from Kemp & David [11]. Reproduced with permission from Dr A David.

hospital did you think you were suffering from a mental disorder?" The validity of this compared with contemporaneous assessments has yet to be tested. Furthermore, using the SAI-E for a wider range of symptoms can be problematic. For example, asking a patient whether an episode of aggression or relationship problems were 'part of their illness' may be moot.

Birchwood Insight Scale

The Birchwood Insight Scale (BIS) [17] is an eight-item self-report insight measure (Figure 7.4), based on the three dimensions in David [12]. Each item is rated on a three-point scale ('agree,' 'disagree,' and 'unsure') with some reverse scored so that, for example, agreement to Question 3 would score 0 while agreement to Question 2 would score 2. The four treatment-related items are combined to preserve the three factors, each of which can score 0–4; hence the range is 0–12.

Commentary on the Birchwood Insight Scale

The authors showed the scale to have good reliability, validity and sensitivity (as measured against other scales and clinical outcomes), as well as being quick and easy to administer. Its test–retest validity over a week is high suggesting it measures a stable and reliable construct. Clearly the weakness of a self-report insight scale is that, at least theoretically, a patient could say, "My stay in hospital is necessary," with the view to conveying good insight, while the astute clinician might regard this as insincere.

Schedule for the assessment of Unawareness of Mental Disorder

The SUMD [18,19] is the most comprehensive, detailed and lengthy of the available insight assessments, with five dimensions that are further divisible by time period (current and retrospective), spanning 74 items. It is a structured interview with each item rated on a five-point Likert scale. Five factors from the assessment of the insight in psychosis by Amador et al [19], overlap in some areas with another model by David [12].

The five factors [19] are an awareness of:
1. having a mental disorder;
2. the effects of medication;
3. the consequences of mental illness;
4. symptoms; and
5. attribution of symptoms to a mental disorder.

As well as splitting David's concept of relabeling symptoms into two (awareness and attribution), the Amador model adds a factor for awareness of consequences, and focuses on awareness of treatment effects rather than need for treatment; it also has a temporal component, so all factors can be split into past and present.

Commentary on the Schedule for the assessment of Unawareness of Mental Disorder

The SUMD has some key differences from the SAI-E and other scales. It measures a temporal dimension, enabling a comparison of a patient's attitude toward current illness as compared with

Figure 7.4 Birchwood Insight Scale

1. Some of my symptoms are made by my mind.
2. I am mentally well.
3. I do not need medication.
4. My stay in hospital is necessary.
5. The doctor is right in prescribing medication for me.
6. I do not need to be seen by a doctor or psychiatrist.
7. If somebody said that I have a nervous or a mental illness then they would be right.
8. None of the unusual things I experience are due to an illness.

Data from Birchwood et al [17]. © 1994, reproduced with permission from John Wiley and Sons.

the past. It also provides a detailed measure of awareness of, and attribution for, a large variety of symptoms. It does not measure patients' attitudes toward treatment. The SUMD may be considered the 'gold standard' for insight assessments and is used most often in the United States. However, due to the detail, it takes considerably longer to administer than other scales and also requires extended training in order to use it reliably.

References

1   David AS. The clinical importance of insight: an overview. In: Amador XF & David AS, eds. *Insight and Psychosis: Awareness of Illness in Schizophrenia and Related Disorders*. 2nd edn. Oxford, UK: Oxford University Press; 2004:359-392.

2   McEvoy JP. The relationship between insight into psychosis and compliance with medications. In: Amador XF & David AS, eds. *Insight and Psychosis: Awareness of Illness in Schizophrenia and Related Disorders*. 2nd edn. Oxford, UK: Oxford University Press; 2004: 311-333.

3   Mintz AR, Dobson KS, Romney DM. Insight in schizophrenia: a meta-analysis. *Schiz Res*. 2003;61:75-88.

4   Aleman A, Agrawal N, Morgan KD, David AS. Insight in psychosis and neuropsychological function: meta-analysis. *Br J Psychiatry*. 2006;189:204-212.

5   Keshavan MS, Rabinowitz J, DeSmedt G, Harvey P.D, Schooler N. Correlates of insight in first episode psychosis. *Schizophr Res*. 2004;70:187-94.

6   Gilleen J, Greenwood K, David AS. Anosognosia in schizophrenia and other neuropsychiatric disorders: similarities and differences. In: Prigatano GP, ed. *The Study of Anosognosia*. Oxford, UK: Oxford University Press; 2010:255-292.

7   Morgan KD, Dazzan P, Morgan C, et al. Insight, grey matter and cognitive function in first-onset psychosis. *Br J Psychiatry*. 2010;197:141-148.

8   Kay SR, Fiszbein A, Opler LA. The Positive and Negative Syndrome Scale (PANSS) for schizophrenia. *Schizophr Bull*. 1987;13:261-276.

9   McEvoy JP, Aland J, Wilson WH, Guy W, Hawkins L. Measuring chronic schizophrenic patients' attitudes toward their illness and treatment. *Hosp Community Psychiatry*. 1981;32:856-858.

10 McEvoy JP, Apperson LJ, Appelbaum PS, et al. Insight in schizophrenia. its relationship to acute psychopathology. *J Nerv Ment Dis*. 1989;177:43-47.

11 Kemp R, David AS. Insight and compliance. In: Blackwell B, ed. *Treatment Compliance and the Therapeutic Alliance*. Amsterdam: Harwood Academic Publishers; 1997:61-86.

12 David AS. Insight and psychosis. *Br J Psychiatry*. 1990;156:798-808.

13 David AS, Buchanan A, Reed A, Almeida O. The assessment of insight in psychosis. *Br J Psychiatry*. 1992;161:599-602.

14 Sanz M, Constable G, Lopez-Ibor I, Kemp R, David A. A comparative study of insight scales and their relationship to psychopathological and clinical variables. *Psychol Med*. 1991;28:437-446.

15 Wiffen BDR, Rabinowitz J, Lex A, David AS. Correlates, change and 'state or trait' properties of insight in schizophrenia. *Schiz Res.* 2010;122:94-103.

16 Owen GS, Richardson G, David AS, Szmukler G, Hayward P, Hotopf M. Mental capacity, diagnosis, and insight in psychiatric inpatients: a cross sectional study. *Psychol Med.* 2009;39:1389-1398.

17 Birchwood M, Smith J, Drury V, Healy J, Macmillan F, Slade M. A self-report Insight Scale for psychosis: reliability, validity and sensitivity to change. *Acta Psychiatr Scand.* 1994;89:62-67.

18 Amador XF, Strauss DH. *The Scale to Assess Unawareness of Mental Disorder (SUMD).* Columbia University and New York State Psychiatric Institute. 1990.

19 Amador XF, Strauss DH, Yale SA, Flaum MM, Endicott J, Gorman JM. Assessment of insight in psychosis. *Am J Psychiatry.* 1993;150:873-879.

8. Assessing adherence to antipsychotic medications

Donald Goff and Julie Kreyenbuhl

Adherence to antipsychotic treatment is essential for achieving optimal therapeutic outcomes in individuals with schizophrenia. However, 60–75% of people with schizophrenia do not take their antipsychotic medications as prescribed [1–3], resulting in exacerbation and relapse of symptoms [4], impaired functioning [5], increased rates of hospitalization [6], and high healthcare costs [7]. The risk of symptom relapse was found to be high even with brief periods of partial nonadherence to antipsychotic treatment early in the course of the illness [8]. Detecting nonadherence to antipsychotics is challenging, and tools for quickly and accurately assessing adherence are needed so that clinicians can readily identify patients likely to be nonadherent and can assess the effectiveness of adherence-enhancing interventions.

Adherence can be evaluated by direct and indirect methods, and no approach is without short-comings. Since no single approach consistently captures every aspect of adherence, multiple approaches should be used [2]. Examples of direct methods include observing patients taking their medications, pill counts, and blood or urine assays. Another example is electronic monitoring, in which a microchip records the date and time of each opening of a pill bottle and which is generally considered the 'gold standard' of adherence assessment. Although these approaches provide relatively objective and valid estimates of medication adherence, widespread implementation in clinical practice has been limited by their greater cost, the greater time commitment required by clinicians, and the relative intrusiveness to patients.

An increasingly common but more indirect approach to assessment of antipsychotic adherence involves analyzing prescription refill patterns from pharmacy records. Although the act of refilling a prescription does not guarantee that medication has been ingested, pharmacy refill patterns have been found to be valid indicators of antipsychotic adherence. Research using pharmacy records has shown that having less than 80% of needed antipsychotics dispensed is associated with increased rates of psychiatric hospitalization and other adverse outcomes in individuals with schizophrenia [6,7].

Due to the limitations of direct methods of adherence assessment, more indirect approaches, primarily self-reports by patients and clinicians, are the most commonly used methods in research [2] and clinical practice. The major limitation of self-reports is that both patients and clinicians often greatly overestimate antipsychotic adherence [9,10]. Despite providing less reliable estimates, indirect approaches are inexpensive and easily implemented in clinical practice as most do not require extensive training to administer.

R. Keefe (ed.), *Guide to Assessment Scales in Schizophrenia*,
DOI: 10.1007/978-1-908517-71-5_8,
© Springer Healthcare, a part of Springer Science+Business Media 2012

Drug Attitude Inventory

One of the earliest developed and most frequently used patient self-report measures designed to predict antipsychotic adherence is the Drug Attitude Inventory (DAI) [11], which measures patients' subjective response to antipsychotic treatment. In a study involving 150 individuals with schizophrenia, the DAI was shown to have adequate internal consistency and test–retest reliability. Validity was evaluated using clinicians' judgment of antipsychotic adherence as the 'gold standard;' the DAI correctly classified 96% of adherent patients and 83% of individuals judged to be nonadherent by their clinicians [11]. The DAI is available in 30- and 10-question versions, the DAI-30 and DAI-10, respectively, consisting of a series of statements rated true or false by the patient, with total scores ranging from –30 (negative subjective response indicating nonadherent behavior) to +30 (positive subjective response indicating adherent behavior) for the DAI-30 and –10 to +10 for DAI-10 (Figure 8.1) [11]. Among the limitations of the DAI is that its validity testing was based on clinicians' judgment of adherence rather than on a more objective measure (eg, electronic monitoring). Furthermore, the scale relies heavily on side effects that may be more relevant to the less frequently prescribed first-generation antipsychotics.

Medication Adherence Rating Scale

The Medication Adherence Rating Scale (MARS) is a ten-item yes/no self-report instrument that also assesses patient attitudes about antipsychotic treatment and the presence of side effects (Figure 8.2) [12]. It was developed from two existing scales, the DAI-30 [11] and the four-item Medication Adherence Questionnaire (MAQ) [13], a brief adherence measure widely used in other

Figure 8.1 The Drug Attitude Inventory

	Patient response	
Statement	False	True
1. For me, the good things about medication outweigh the bad.		
2. I feel weird, like a zombie, on medication.		
3. I take medications of my own free choice.		
4. Medications make me feel more relaxed.		
5. Medication makes me feel tired and sluggish.		
6. I take medication only when I am sick.		
7. I feel more normal on medication.		
8. It is unnatural for my mind and body to be controlled by medications.		
9. My thoughts are clearer on medication.		
10. By staying on medications, I can prevent getting sick.		

If you would like to use the DAI-30 or DAI-10 or obtain further information please contact the copyright holder. Data from Hogan et al [11]. ©1987, reproduced with permission from the Oxford University Press.

areas of medicine. Total scores on the MARS range from 0 (low likelihood of medication adherence) to 10 (high likelihood). Although initial work showed the MARS to be reliable and valid [12], concerns were raised because it was evaluated in a diagnostically heterogeneous sample and validated with blood levels of mood stabilizer medications rather than antipsychotics. A subsequent study in individuals with schizophrenia disorders showed lower internal consistency than initially reported. Furthermore, only the four items corresponding to the MAQ were significantly correlated with clinician ratings of antipsychotic adherence, leading the investigators to conclude that the four MAQ items may be preferred over the MARS total score as a measure of medication adherence behavior [14]. The MARS shares one of the major limitations of the DAI in not having its validity tested against a more objective measure of adherence.

Brief Evaluation of Medication Influences and Beliefs

The Brief Evaluation of Medication Influences and Beliefs (BEMIB) (Figure 8.3) [15] is another patient self-report scale consisting of eight statements addressing the five domains of the health beliefs model, which has been shown to correlate with medication adherence:

1. Benefits of treatment.
2. Risks of illness.
3. Costs of treatment, including side effects and other inconveniences.
4. Barriers to treatment.
5. Cues to act (ie, medication management strategies).

Responses to the eight statements are made on a Likert-type scale ranging from 1 (completely disagree) to 5 (completely agree); one or more ratings of '1' or '2' is considered to be the threshold for nonadherence. The reliability and validity of the BEMIB was evaluated in 63 outpatients with

Figure 8.2 Medication Adherence Rating Scale

Please respond to the following statements by marking in the column the response which best describes your behavior or the attitude you have held toward your medication in the past week.

		Yes	No
1.	Do you ever forget to take your medication?		
2.	Are you careless at times about taking your medicine?		
3.	When you feel better, do you sometimes stop taking your medicine?		
4.	Sometimes if you feel worse when you take the medicine, do you stop taking it?		
5.	I take my medication only when I am sick.		
6.	It is unnatural for my mind and body to be controlled by medication.		
7.	My thoughts are clearer on medication.		
8.	By staying on medication I can prevent myself getting sick.		
9.	I feel weird, like a 'zombie,' on medication.		

Data from Thompson et al [12]. ©2000, reproduced with permission from Elsevier.

Figure 8.3 The Brief Evaluation of Medication Influences and Beliefs

My antipsychotic medication:

The following questions involve your antipsychotic medication. There are no right or wrong answers, but your honest response is important. Please respond to the following statements regarding your medication by circling the answer that best matches how you agree or disagree.

1. Taking my antipsychotic medication makes me feel better

1	2	3	4	5
Completely disagree	Disagree	Undecided (neither agree nor disagree)	Agree	Completely agree

2. Taking my antipsychotic medication helps prevent me being hospitalized

1	2	3	4	5
Completely disagree	Disagree	Undecided (neither agree nor disagree)	Agree	Completely agree

3. Side effects from my antipsychotic medication bother me

1	2	3	4	5
Completely disagree	Disagree	Undecided (neither agree nor disagree)	Agree	Completely agree

4. I have a system that helps me (eg, pill box, medication calendar, someone giving me my medication) that helps me to remember taking my antipsychotic medication

1	2	3	4	5
Completely disagree	Disagree	Undecided (neither agree nor disagree)	Agree	Completely agree

5. Taking my antipsychotic medication is difficult to remember every day

1	2	3	4	5
Completely disagree	Disagree	Undecided (neither agree nor disagree)	Agree	Completely agree

6. Getting my antipsychotic medication from the hospital or pharmacy is not a problem

1	2	3	4	5
Completely disagree	Disagree	Undecided (neither agree nor disagree)	Agree	Completely agree

7. I am supported by my family, friends, and doctors to take my antipsychotic medication

1	2	3	4	5
Completely disagree	Disagree	Undecided (neither agree nor disagree)	Agree	Completely agree

8. I have a psychiatric disorder that antipsychotic medication improves

1	2	3	4	5
Completely disagree	Disagree	Undecided (neither agree nor disagree)	Agree	Completely agree

Data from Dolder et al [15]. ©2004, reproduced with permission from Lippincott Williams.

schizophrenia and other psychotic disorders in which antipsychotic prescription refill patterns were used as the reference adherence measurement. Although those meeting criteria for nonadherence on the BEMIB had significantly larger gaps in antipsychotic therapy than those not meeting the criteria, classification of nonadherence according to the BEMIB and antipsychotic refill patterns were only in agreement in 67% of cases. In addition, only a moderate level of internal consistency reliability for the BEMIB was found. The BEMIB is also limited by being evaluated in middle-aged to older outpatient veterans whose medication adherence behaviors may not generalize to other individuals with schizophrenia [15].

Brief Adherence Rating Scale

Although patients' beliefs and attitudes toward antipsychotic medications are important considerations in shared decision-making around treatment and have been shown to be predictive of adherence behaviors, none of the aforementioned scales assess medication-taking behaviors or provide estimates of actual levels of adherence. The recently developed Brief Adherence Rating Scale (BARS) [16] addresses several of the limitations of previous adherence assessments. The BARS is a four-item clinician-administered scale, in which three items are used to evaluate the patient's knowledge of their medication regimen and the frequency of missed or altered doses. Based on these responses, the clinician marks on a visual analog scale that ranges from 0% to 100% the estimated proportion of antipsychotic doses taken by the patient in the past month (Figure 8.4) [16]. The reliability and validity of the BARS was evaluated in 61 individuals with schizophrenia disorders, and it is the only antipsychotic adherence scale to be evaluated against electronic adherence monitoring as the reference standard. The BARS was demonstrated to have moderate to high internal consistency and test–retest reliability. Although a significant positive relationship was found between BARS ratings and electronic adherence monitoring, agreement between the two adherence assessments only occurred in 64% of cases [17]. However, greater BARS adherence was found to be significantly related to lower symptom severity as measured by the Positive and Negative Syndrome Scale (PANSS) total score and positive symptom subscale score. Among the strengths of the BARS is that it is simple, brief, and efficient in its administration, and provides an estimate of adherence reported as a percentage (0–100%) of medication taken, which is the method that is recommended by experts [18].

Overall, a comprehensive approach to the assessment of antipsychotic adherence, which includes utilizing direct measures when available and understanding patients' positive and negative attitudes toward medications, is likely the best strategy for predicting patients at risk for poor adherence and guiding the choice of interventions to improve adherence.

Figure 8.4 The Brief Adherence Rating Scale

Patient identification:		Date:
The following information is obtained by the clinician:		
1. How many pills of _____ (name of antipsychotic) did the doctor tell you to take each day?		
2. Over the month since your last visit with me, on how many days did you **not take** your _____ (name of antipsychotic)?	Few if any (<7)	
	7–13	
	14–20	
	Most (>20)	
3. Over the month since your last visit with me, how many days did you **take less than** the prescribed number of pills of your _____ (name of antipsychotic)?	Always/almost always = 1 (76–100% of the time)	
	Usually = 2 (51–75% of the time)	
	Sometimes = 3 (26–50% of the time)	
Note: 1 = Poor adherence 4 = Good adherence	Never/almost never = 4 (0–25% of the time)	

Please place a single vertical line on the dotted line below that you believe best describes, out of the prescribed antipsychotic medication (_____) doses, the proportion of doses taken by the patient in the past month.

None	Half	All
0% 10% 20% 30% 40%	50% 60% 70%	80% 90% 100%

Response struck on above line (%) =	
Rater's initials:	

Data from Byerly et al [16]. ©2008, reproduced with permission from Elsevier.

References

1 Valenstein M, Ganoczy D, McCarthy JF, Myra Kim H, Lee TA, Blow FC. Antipsychotic adherence over time among patients receiving treatment for schizophrenia: a retrospective review. *J Clin Psychiatry.* 2006;67:1542-1550.

2 Velligan DI, Lam YW, Glahn DC, et al. Defining and assessing adherence to oral antipsychotics: a review of the literature. *Schizophr Bull.* 2006;32:724-742.

3 Byerly MJ, Nakonezny PA, Lescouflair E. Antipsychotic medication adherence in schizophrenia. *Psychiatr Clin North Am.* 2007;30:437-452.

4 Lacro JP, Dunn LB, Dolder CR, Leckband SG, Jeste DV. Prevalence of and risk factors for medication nonadherence in patients with schizophrenia: a comprehensive review of recent literature. *J Clin Psychiatry.* 2002;63:892-909.

5 Ascher-Svanum H, Faries DE, Zhu B, et al. Medication adherence and long-term functional outcomes in the treatment of schizophrenia in usual care. *J Clin Psychiatry.* 2006;67:453-460.

6   Valenstein M, Copeland LA, Blow FC, et al. Pharmacy data identify poorly adherent patients with schizophrenia at increased risk for admission. *Med Care*. 2002;40:630-639.

7   Gilmer TP, Dolder CR, Lacro JP, et al. Adherence to treatment with antipsychotic medication and health care costs among Medicaid beneficiaries with schizophrenia. *Am J Psychiatry*. 2004;161:692-699.

8   Subotnik KL, Nuechterlein KH, Ventura J, et al. Risperidone nonadherence and return of positive symptoms in the early course of schizophrenia. *Am J Psychiatry*. 2011;168:286-292.

9   Byerly MJ, Thompson A, Carmody T, et al. Validity of electronically monitored medication adherence and conventional adherence measures in schizophrenia. *Psychiatr Serv*. 2007;58:844-847.

10 Velligan DI, Wang M, Diamond P, et al. Relationships among subjective and objective measures of adherence to oral antipsychotic medications. *Psychiatr Serv*. 2007;58:1187-1192.

11 Hogan TP, Awad AG, Eastwood MR. A self-report scale predictive of drug compliance in schizophrenics: reliability and discriminative validity. *Psychol Med*. 1983;13:177-118.

12 Thompson K, Kulkarni J, Sergejew AA. Reliability and validity of a new Medication Adherence Rating Scale (MARS) for the psychoses. *Schizophr Res*. 2000;42:241-247.

13 Morisky DE, Green LW, Levine DM. Concurrent and predictive validity of a self-reported measure of medication adherence. *Med Care*. 1986;24:67-74.

14 Fialko L, Garety PA, Kuipers E, et al. A large-scale validation study of the Medication Adherence Rating Scale (MARS). *Schizophr Res*. 2008;100:53-59.

15 Dolder CR, Lacro JP, Warren KA, et al. Brief evaluation of medication influences and beliefs: development and testing of a brief scale for medication adherence. *J Clin Psychopharmacol*. 2004;24:404-409.

16 Byerly MJ, Nakonezny PA, Rush AJ. The Brief Adherence Rating Scale (BARS) validated against electronic monitoring in assessing the antipsychotic medication adherence of outpatients with schizophrenia and schizoaffective disorder. *Schizophr Res*. 2008;100:60-69.

17 Byerly MJ, Thompson A, Carmody T, et al. Validity of electronically monitored medication adherence and conventional adherence measures in schizophrenia. *Psychiatr Serv*. 2007;8:844-847.

18 Velligan DI, Weiden PJ, Sajatovic M, et al. Strategies for addressing adherence problems in patients with serious and persistent mental illness: recommendations from the expert consensus guidelines. *J Psychiatr Pract*. 2010;16:306-324.

9. Clinical assessment scales in substance use disorders

Ashwin A Patkar and Jonathan C Lee

The prevalence of substance use disorders (SUD) is more prevalent in patients with schizophrenia than in the general population, and therefore organized assessment of SUD in this patient group is important in both clinical practice and in research [1]. Reliable and valid measures permit early identification of SUD and evaluation of interventions. In this chapter, we describe widely used assessment instruments for SUD.

Diagnostic instruments

The Mini-International Neuropsychiatric Interview
The Mini-International Neuropsychiatric Interview (MINI) is a brief psychiatric interview that can be completed in approximately 15 minutes [2,3]. The MINI is comprised of several modules that yield diagnoses consistent with the *Diagnostic and Statistical Manual of Mental Disorders* (DSM-IV) [4] Axis I disorders including substance abuse and dependence. There is an additional module that assesses dependence specifically to a variety of prescription drugs, rather than 'street' drugs [5].

Composite International Diagnostic Interview
The Composite International Diagnostic Interview (CIDI) [6] is a comprehensive, structured interview developed by the World Health Organization (WHO). It takes approximately 2 hours to complete and assesses 22 DSM-IV and the *International Statistical Classification of Diseases and Related Health Problems – 10th Revision* (ICD-10) [7] diagnoses, including SUD. For each SUD, the CIDI elicits information that is useful for treatment planning such as pattern and course of substance use. It is used in epidemiological studies as well as for research and clinical purposes.

The Structured Clinical Interview for DSM-IV Axis I
The Structured Clinical Interview for DSM-IV Axis I (SCID-I) [8] is a semi-structured interview that provides lifetime and current diagnoses for major DSM-IV Axis I disorders including SUD. Administration can take hours depending upon the number of modules. The SCID is often considered the 'gold standard' in determining the accuracy of clinical diagnoses in research [9]. The reliability for diagnoses of alcohol and other substance use disorders is high, with kappa values ranging from 0.65 to 1.0 [10].

R. Keefe (ed.), *Guide to Assessment Scales in Schizophrenia*,
DOI: 10.1007/978-1-908517-71-5_9,
© Springer Healthcare, a part of Springer Science+Business Media 2012

Screening instruments

Screening instruments to detect the presence of alcohol-use disorders include the CAGE Questionnaire [11,12], the name of which is an acronym of its four questions (Figure 9.1), and the Alcohol Use Disorders Identification Test (AUDIT) [13] (Figure 9.2) [14].

The CAGE Questionnaire
The CAGE Questionnaire is an internationally used instrument to identify problem drinking [11]. It has four questions that require a yes/no response and takes a minute to complete. The CAGE is most effective when used as part of a general health history [15]. The CAGE Questionnaire Adapted to Include Drugs (CAGE-AID) is a modified version of CAGE to screen for both alcohol and illicit drug use disorders [12]. For the CAGE and CAGE-AID, two of four affirmative answers are considered a positive screen that requires further evaluation.

The Alcohol Use Disorders Identification Test
The AUDIT was developed by the WHO to screen for excessive drinking. It can be used in a variety of health settings and provides a framework for intervention to help drinkers reduce or cease alcohol consumption and thereby avoid the harmful consequences of their drinking. An AUDIT score of 8 or more is associated with harmful drinking; a score of 13 or more in women, and 15 or more in men, is suggestive of alcohol dependence [14]. Positive screens for the CAGE, CAGE-AID, and AUDIT should be followed by evaluation to determine the presence of DSM-IV SUD [4].

Figure 9.1 The CAGE Questionnaire

- Have you ever felt you should **c**ut down on your drinking?
- Have people **a**nnoyed you by criticizing your drinking?
- Have you ever felt bad or **g**uilty about your drinking?
- Have you ever had a drink first thing in the morning to steady your nerves or get rid of a hangover (**e**ye-opener)?

Score: /4
2/4 or greater = positive CAGE, further evaluation is indicated

CAGE Questionnaire Adapted to Include Drugs

1. Have you felt you ought to cut down on your drinking or drug use?
2. Have people annoyed you by criticizing your drinking or drug use?
3. Have you felt bad or guilty about your drinking or drug use?
4. Have you ever had a drink or used drugs first thing in the morning to steady your nerves or to get rid of a hangover (eye-opener)?

Score: /4
2/4 or greater = positive CAGE, further evaluation is indicated

Two of four affirmative answers are considered a positive screen. CAGE Questionnaire data from Ewing [11], © 2008, American Medical Association. CAGE Questionnaire Adapted to Include Drugs data from Brown & Rounds [12], reprinted with permission from the Wisconsin Medical Journal.

Figure 9.2 Alcohol Use Disorders Identification Test

1.   How often do you have a drink containing alcohol?

- Never
- Monthly or less
- 2–4 times a month
- 2 or 3 times a week
- 4 or more times a week

2.   How many standard drinks containing alcohol do you have on a typical day when drinking?

- 1 or 2
- 3 or 4
- 5 or 6
- 7–9
- 10 or more

3.   How often do you have six or more drinks on one occasion?

- Never
- Less than monthly
- Monthly
- Weekly
- Daily or almost daily

4.   During the past year, how often have you found that you were not able to stop drinking once you had started?

- Never
- Less than monthly
- Monthly
- Weekly
- Daily or almost daily

5.   During the past year, how often have you failed to do what was normally expected of you because of drinking?

- Never
- Less than monthly
- Monthly
- Weekly
- Daily or almost daily

6.   During the past year, how often have you needed a drink in the morning to get yourself going after a heavy drinking session?

- Never
- Less than monthly
- Monthly
- Weekly
- Daily or almost daily

7.   During the past year, how often have you had a feeling of guilt or remorse after drinking?

- Never
- Less than monthly
- Monthly
- Weekly
- Daily or almost daily

(continues overleaf).

Figure 9.2 Alcohol Use Disorders Identification Test (continued)

8. During the past year, have you been unable to remember what happened the night before because you had been drinking?
• Never
• Less than monthly
• Monthly
• Weekly
• Daily or almost daily

9. Have you or someone else been injured as a result of your drinking?
• No
• Yes, but not in the past year
• Yes, during the past year

10. Has a relative or friend, doctor or other health worker been concerned about your drinking or suggested you cut down?
• No
• Yes, but not in the past year
• Yes, during the past year

Scoring the AUDIT

Scores for questions 1–8 range from 0 to 4, with responses of the first option (eg, 'Never' or '1 or 2') scoring 0, the second scoring 1, the third scoring 2, the fourth scoring 3, and responses of the fifth option scoring 4. For questions 9 and 10, which only have three responses, the scoring is 0 for 'Never', 2 for 'Yes, but not in the past year', and 4 for 'Yes, during the past year'. A score of 8 or more is associated with harmful or hazardous drinking, a score of 13 or more in women, and 15 or more in men, is likely to indicate alcohol dependence.

(continued). Data from Saunders et al [14]. ©2001 World Health Organization.

The Drug Abuse Screening Test

The Drug Abuse Screening Test (DAST) [16] is a 28-item self-report instrument to screen for drug-related problems [17]. The DAST yields a quantitative score for the degree of consequences related to drug abuse. It takes 5 minutes to administer and may be given in questionnaire, interview, or computerized formats. Subsequent versions include a 20-item DAST (DAST-20) and an abbreviated ten-item version (DAST-10) that have comparable reliability and validity to the original version.

Withdrawal rating scales

The Clinical Institute Withdrawal Assessment for Alcohol (CIWA-A) is used to assess the severity of alcohol withdrawal. There is a shortened version known as CIWA-A Revised (CIWA-Ar) [17] that takes about 5 minutes to complete. For the CIWA-Ar, a score of more than 18 indicates severe withdrawal, 10–18 moderate withdrawal, and 9 or less indicates mild withdrawal [19].

Validated opioid withdrawal scales include the following:

- Clinical Opiate Withdrawal Scale (COWS) [20];
- 10-item Short Opiate Withdrawal Scale [21];

- 16-item Subjective Opiate Withdrawal Scale;
- 13-item Objective Opioid Withdrawal Scale (OOWS) [22].

A COWS score of 5–12 indicates mild opioid withdrawal, 13–24 moderate withdrawal, 25–36 moderately severe withdrawal, and more than 36 indicates severe withdrawal.

Addiction Severity Index

The Addiction Severity Index (ASI) is a 45-minute, semi-structured interview that is widely used in substance abuse treatment settings [23,24]. The ASI collects data regarding the seven functional domains: medical, employment/support, drug and alcohol use, legal, family history, family/social relationships, and psychiatric problems. It yields a severity score and a composite score. The composite scores are useful for summarizing changes in patient status, which can be utilized in treatment outcome studies. Shorter versions (ASI-Lite) have been developed to facilitate adoption in clinical settings [25].

Readiness-to-Change Scale

The Readiness-to-Change Scale [26] is used to evaluate a person's readiness or motivation to change. This assessment promotes identification and discussion of perceived barriers to change. The scale can provide the basis for motivation-based interventions to elicit behavior change in SUD [27].

Validity and reliability issues in self-report scales

Validity issues in self-report scales can be due to exaggeration or minimization of the severity or frequency of symptoms. The participant may also neglect to report symptoms and/or manipulate information for secondary gain. Results can be skewed by participants' social desirability biases and/or lack of respondents' biases. Therefore administration of rating scales should be accompanied by a good clinical evaluation. Nevertheless, several scales have demonstrated good reliability, validity, and acceptance in research settings and are gaining wider acceptance in clinical settings to inform treatment planning.

References

1 Volkow ND. Substance use disorders in schizophrenia – clinical implications of comorbidity. *Schizophr Bull.* 2009;35:469-472.
2 Medical Outcome Systems. The Mini International Neuropsychiatric Interview version 6.0 (M.I.N.I. 6.0). Available at: www.medical-outcomes.com/index.php. Accessed April 2, 2012.
3 Sheehan DV, Lecrubier Y, Sheehan KH, et al. The Mini-International Neuropsychiatric Interview (M.I.N.I.): the development and validation of a structured diagnostic psychiatric interview for DSM-IV and ICD-10. *J Clin Psychiatry.* 1998;59:22-33.
4 American Psychiatric Association. *Diagnostic and Statistical Manual of Mental Disorders.* 4th edn. Text Revision. Washington, DC: American Psychiatric Association; 2000.

5 Patton DP, Lemaire J, Friesen K. Still without shelter: a description of issues faced by street youth in Winnipeg in 2007. Addictions Foundation of Manitoba; October 2008.

6 World Health Organization. The WHO Composite International Diagnostic Interview (CIDI). Available at: www.hcp.med.harvard.edu/wmhcidi. Accessed April 2, 2012.

7 World Health Organization. International Statistical Classification of Diseases and Related Health Problems 10th Revision. Available at: apps.who.int/classifications/apps/icd/icd10online. Accessed April 2, 2012.

8 First MB. Structured Clinical Interview for DSM Disorders (SCID). Available at: www.scid4.org. Accessed April 2, 2012.

9 Shear MK, Greeno C, Kang, J, et al. Diagnosis of nonpsychotic patients in community clinics. *Am J Psychiatry*. 2000;157:581-587.

10 First MB. What is the reliability of the SCID-I? Available at: www.scid4.org/psychometric/scidl_reliability.html. Accessed April 2, 2012.

11 Ewing JA. Detecting alcoholism: The CAGE Questionnaire. *JAMA*.1984;252:1905-1907.

12 Brown RL, Rounds LA. Conjoint screening questionnaires for alcohol and drug abuse. *Wisc Med J*. 1995;94:135-140.

13 Ries RI, Fiellin DA, Miller SC, Saitz R. *Principles of Addiction Medicine*. 4th edn. Philadelphia, PA: Lippincott Williams & Wilkins; 2009:267-294.

14 Saunders JB, Aasland OG, Babor TF, et al. Development of the alcohol use disorders identification test (AUDIT): WHO collaborative project on early detection of persons with harmful alcohol consumption-II. *Addiction*. 1993;88:791-803.

15 Steinweg DL, Worth H. Alcoholism: the keys to the CAGE. *Am J Med*. 1993;94:520-523.

16 Tepp AV. Substance Abuse Screening Instrument. Available at: www.drtepp.com/pdf/substance_abuse.pdf. Accessed April 2, 2012.

17 Gavin DR, Ross HE, Skinner HA. Diagnostic validity of the Drug Abuse Screening Test in the assessment of DSM-III drug disorders. *Br J Addict*. 1989;84:301-307.

18 Sullivan JT, Sykora K, Schneiderman J, et al. Clinical Institute Withdrawal Assessment of Alcohol Scale, revised. Available at: umem.org/files/uploads/1104212257_CIWA-Ar.pdf. Accessed April 2, 2012.

19 Sullivan JT, Sykora K, Schneiderman J, et al. Assessment of alcohol withdrawal: The revised Clinical Institute Withdrawal Assessment for Alcohol scale (CIWA-Ar). *Br J Addict*. 1989;84:1353-1357.

20 Wesson Dr, Ling W. The Clinical Opiate Withdrawal Scale (COWS). *J Psychoactive Drugs*. 2003;25:253-259.

21 Gossop M. The development of a Short Opiate Withdrawal Scale (SOWS). *Addict Behav*. 1990;15:487-490.

22 Handelsman L, Cochrane KJ, Aronson MJ, et al. Two new rating scales for opiate withdrawal. *Am J Drug Alcohol Abuse*. 1987;13:293-308.

23 Treatment Research Institute. The Addiction Severity Index. Available at: www.tresearch.org/asi.htm. Accessed April 2, 2012.

24 McLellan AT, Cacciola JS, Alterman AI, et al. The Addiction Severity Index at 25: origins, contributions and transitions. *Am J Addict*. 2006;15:113-124.

25 Addiction Severity Index – Lite Version (ASI-Lite). Available at: www.who.int/substance_abuse/research_tools/addictionseverity/en/index.html. Accessed April 2, 2012.

26 Adult Meducation. Readiness-to-Change Ruler. Available at: www.adultmeducation.com/AssessmentTools_3.html. Accessed April 2, 2012.

27 Zimmerman GL, Olsen CG, Bosworth MF. A 'stages of change' approach to helping patients change behavior. *Am Fam Physician*. 2000;61:1409-1416.

10. Medical comorbidities

Joseph P McEvoy

The mortality rate of individuals with schizophrenia is two to three times higher than that of age-, race-, and gender-matched controls; individuals with schizophrenia die, on average, 15–30 years earlier than their peers [1]. They are three times as likely to be obese and twice as likely to have the metabolic syndrome; the metabolic syndrome confers a five- or sixfold increased likelihood of diabetes mellitus and a three- to sixfold increase in mortality from cardiovascular disease [2].

A poor diet, sedentary lifestyle, and smoking contribute to these metabolic and cardiovascular problems. In addition, since the availability of the original atypical antipsychotic medications, the gap in mortality between patients with schizophrenia and the general population has widened and the incidence of diabetes mellitus has accelerated, which may be associated with the direct effects of these agents on metabolism [2].

Individuals with schizophrenia, especially those with comorbid substance abuse disorders, are also at elevated risk for infectious disease. Prevalence rates for hepatitis B virus and hepatitis C virus are approximately 20% in individuals with schizophrenia, 5 and 11 times the general population rates, respectively [2]. Among high-risk, drug-using individuals (those who share needles, engage in unprotected sex, or trade sex for money or drugs) with schizophrenia rates of positive tests for human immunodeficiency virus (HIV) may be as high as 20% [2].

The first-generation antipsychotics and the second-generation antipsychotics risperidone and paliperidone, produce substantial elevations in prolactin, resulting in physical and behavioral alterations [3]. Direct consequences of sustained prolactin elevation induced by antipsychotic medication include breast engorgement and tenderness and galactorrhea in men and women. Indirect consequences of hyperprolactinemia in women (via suppression of estrogen levels) include oligomenorrhea and amenorrhea, erratic or absent ovulation, and sexual dysfunction [4], as well as reduced bone mineral density [5]. In men, prolactin-induced suppression of testosterone levels results in sexual dysfunction.

Individuals with schizophrenia often fail to seek health care [6]. They are less capable than the general population of identifying and interpreting physical signs, and less capable of caring for their medical illnesses. In many cases, the only contact an individual with schizophrenia has with the health care system is through the mental health care team. For this reason, mental health clinicians are at the forefront of physical health care for patients with schizophrenia [7].

R. Keefe (ed.), *Guide to Assessment Scales in Schizophrenia*,
DOI: 10.1007/978-1-908517-71-5_10,
© Springer Healthcare, a part of Springer Science+Business Media 2012

Setting the baseline

All patients should have their weight, pulse rate, and blood pressure recorded when first admitted to a clinic and at least yearly thereafter. A prolactin level, hemoglobin A1c, and lipid profile (total-, high-density lipoproteins, and low-density lipoproteins cholesterol, and triglyceride levels), and C-reactive protein (CRP) levels should be obtained at similar intervals.

Starting new antipsychotic medications

Weight should be recorded at least monthly after a new antipsychotic medication is started. If the medication has a known liability to produce metabolic effects, hemoglobin A1c, a lipid profile, and CRP levels should be obtained after 1 and 2 months. If the medication has a known liability to produce prolactin elevations, a prolactin level should be obtained after 1 month. The Antipsychotic Medication Monitoring Form can be copied and placed in the patient's chart to record these measures (Figure 10.1).

Health issues for women

The health checklist for women can be copied and placed in the chart of a patient with schizophrenia to guide monitoring (Figure 10.2).

Figure 10.1 New Antipsychotic Medication Monitoring Form

Medication:		Start date:	
	Baseline	**1 month**	**2 months**
	Interval date:	Interval date:	Interval date:
Height			
Weight			
Blood pressure			
Pulse			
Prolactin level			
Hemoglobin A1c			
Triglycerides			
Total cholesterol			
LDL cholesterol			
HDL cholesterol			
C-reactive protein			

HDL, high-density lipoproteins; LDL, low-density lipoproteins.

Human papillomavirus immunization

The human papillomavirus (HPV) immunization vaccine protects against genital warts, cervical cancer, and other less common cancers. The vaccines are given in three shots; it is important to get all three shots to have the best protection. The vaccines are most effective when given at 11–12 years of age, but can be usefully administered to women up to 26 years of age who did not get any or all of the shots when they were younger [8].

Sexually transmitted diseases

Female patients with schizophrenia should be advised that their chances of being infected with sexually transmitted diseases (STDs) are reduced by: being in a monogamous sexual relationship, limiting the number of sex partners, if their partner has had no or few prior sex partners, and by using condoms with each sexual encounter, from start to finish.

Figure 10.2 Women's health checklist

Human papillomavirus (HPV) immunization		
Done: (Y/N)	Indicated, not done: (Y/N)	Not indicated: (Y/N)
Date:	Date:	Date:
Urine testing for chlamydia and gonorrhea		
Done: (Y/N)	Indicated, not done: (Y/N)	Not indicated: (Y/N)
Date:	Date:	Date:
Results (date):		
Testing for syphilis, hepatitis B virus, hepatitis C virus, and HIV		
Done: (Y/N)	Indicated, not done: (Y/N)	Not indicated: (Y/N)
Date:	Date:	Date:
Results (date):		
Birth control		
Done: (Y/N)	Indicated, not done: (Y/N)	Not indicated: (Y/N)
Date:	Date:	Date:
Method:		
Pap screening		
Done: (Y/N)	Indicated, not done: (Y/N)	Not indicated: (Y/N)
Date:	Date:	Date:
Results (date):		
Mammography		
Done: (Y/N)	Indicated, not done: (Y/N)	Not indicated: (Y/N)
Date:	Date:	Date:
Results (date):		

Pap, Papanicolaou.

Urine testing for chlamydia and gonorrhea should be done annually for sexually active women ≤25 years old, and for women >25 years old who are at risk (eg, have had multiple sexual partners or starting a relationship with a new sexual partner) [9].

Testing for syphilis, hepatitis B virus, hepatitis C virus, and HIV should be done once when a woman is first seen for treatment and then yearly for women at risk (those who test positive for chlamydia or gonorrhea, or who have more than one sexual partner over the prior year).

Birth control

While the overall rate of pregnancy in women with schizophrenia of child-bearing age is lower than in the general population, the percentage of pregnancies that are unwanted is higher than that in the general population [10]. Contraceptive counseling to women and their partners is an important part of comprehensive care for women with serious and persistent mental illness. The majority of women with schizophrenia smoke, are overweight, or have diabetes, migraine, cardiovascular disease, or a family history of breast cancer; these women should be offered nonhormonal contraception.

Women with more than one sexual partner should be advised on barrier methods (which protect from STDs) in addition to any other contraceptive measures they are using.

Long-lasting contraceptive methods, such as intrauterine devices, progesterone depot injections, or tubal ligation are reasonable options for women having no wish to further expand their families [10].

Cancer screening

Women with psychosis are more than five times less likely to receive adequate Papanicolaou (Pap) screening compared with the general population despite their increased rates of smoking and increased number of primary care visits [11]. Pap screening should be done every 2 years for women age 21–30 years old, and every 3 years for women over 30 years of age whose previous three tests have been normal.

Mammography

At the Mayo Clinic a three-tiered approach is used [12]:

- Breast health awareness, which includes a woman becoming familiar with her breasts in order to identify breast abnormalities or changes, and to inform her doctor of any changes that may need further evaluation.
- Clinical breast exam performed by a health care provider and recommended annually beginning at age 40 years.
- Screening mammography every 2 years beginning at age 40 years.

Health issues for men

The health checklist for men can be copied and placed in the chart of a patient with schizophrenia to guide monitoring (Figure 10.3). Urine testing for chlamydia and gonorrhea, and testing for syphilis, hepatitis B and C viruses, and HIV should be undertaken with the same timings as previously discussed for female patients. Discussion of safe-sex practices and condom use should be undertaken yearly. Many psycho-active medications can impair sexual functioning in men [13]. This should be addressed at least yearly.

Prostate cancer screening

Prostate cancer screening should be offered to all men aged 50 years or older and men with at least a 10-year life expectancy. Annual screening has been the standard. If there is a higher risk for prostate cancer, such as family history of prostate cancer or if the patient is of African heritage, screening should be offered from age 40 years. Furthermore, there may be a benefit in offering a baseline prostate-specific antigen (PSA) test for men between 40 and 49 years of age to establish future prostate cancer risk. Initial screening should include digital rectal examination and PSA [14].

Figure 10.3 Men's health checklist

Urine testing for chlamydia and gonorrhea		
Done: (Y/N)	Indicated, not done: (Y/N)	Not indicated: (Y/N)
Date:	Date:	Date:
Results (date):		
Testing for syphilis, hepatitis B virus, hepatitis C virus, and HIV		
Done: (Y/N)	Indicated, not done: (Y/N)	Not indicated: (Y/N)
Date:	Date:	Date:
Results (date):		
Discussion of condom use		
Done: (Y/N)	Indicated, not done: (Y/N)	Not indicated: (Y/N)
Date:	Date:	Date:
Discussion of sexual functioning		
Done: (Y/N)	Indicated, not done: (Y/N)	Not indicated: (Y/N)
Date:	Date:	Date:
Prostate cancer screening (PSA and digital rectal examination)		
Done: (Y/N)	Indicated, not done: (Y/N)	Not indicated: (Y/N)
Date:	Date:	Date:
Results (date):		

References

1 Black DW. Mortality in schizophrenia – the Iowa record-linkage study: a comparison with general population mortality. *Psychosomatics*. 1988;29:55-60.

2 De Hert M, Correll CU, Bobes J, et al. Physical illness in patients with severe mental disorders. I. Prevalence, impact of medications and disparities in health care. *World Psychiatry*. 2011;10:52-77.

3 Inder WJ, Castle D. Antipsychotic-induced hyperprolactinaemia. *Aust N Z J Psychiatry*. 2011; 45:830-837.

4 Bushe CJ, Bradley A, Pendlebury J. A review of hyperprolactinaemia and severe mental illness: are there implications for clinical biochemistry? *Ann Clin Biochem*. 2010; 47:292-300.

5 Graham SM, Howgate D, Anderson W, et al. Risk of osteoporosis and fracture incidence in patients on antipsychotic medication. *Expert Opin Drug Saf*. 2011;10: 575-602.

6 Lord O, Malone D, Mitchell AJ. Receipt of preventive medical care and medical screening for patients with mental illness: a comparative analysis. *Gen Hosp Psychiatry*. 2010;32:519-543.

7 De Hert M, Cohen D, Bobes J, et al. Physical illness in patients with severe mental disorders. II. Barriers to care, monitoring and treatment guidelines, plus recommendations at the system and individual level. *World Psychiatry*. 2011;10:138-151.

8 Centers for Disease Control and Prevention. Human papillomavirus (HPV). Available at: www.cdc.gov/std/hpv. Accessed April 2, 2012.

9 US Preventive Services Task Force. Screening for chlamydial infection. Available at: www.uspreventiveservicestaskforce.org/uspstf/uspschlm.htm. Accessed April 2, 2012.

10 Seeman MV, Ross R. Prescribing contraceptives for women with schizophrenia. *J Psychiatr Pract*. 2011;17:258-269.

11 Tilbrook D, Polsky J, Lofters A. Are women with psychosis receiving adequate cervical cancer screening? *Can Fam Physician*. 2010;56:358-363.

12 Mayo Clinic. Mammogram. Available at: www.mayoclinic.com/health/mammogram-guidelines/AN02052. Accessed April 2, 2012.

13 Beckman TJ, Litin SC. Clinical pearls in men's health. *Mayo Clin Proc*. 2010;85:668-673.

14 Izawa JI, Klotz L, Siemens DR, et al. Prostate cancer screening: Canadian guidelines 2011. *Can Urol Assoc J*. 2011;5:235-240.